Discarded by
Hollywood Library

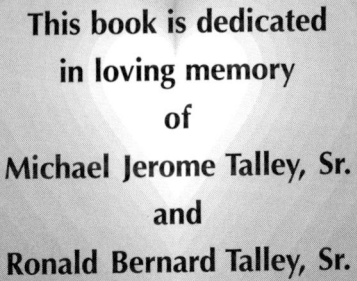

This book is dedicated
in loving memory
of
Michael Jerome Talley, Sr.
and
Ronald Bernard Talley, Sr.

I miss you dearly.
You will always be
in my heart.

ACKNOWLEDGEMENTS

I thank my Heavenly Father for allowing me the opportunity to write this book. You have brought me from a mighty long way. I thank you Lord for healing my body of cancer, and I thank You for showing me what You would have me to do.

I thank my husband, Floyd, for sharing the journey of developing this book with me.

I thank my children, Alisa, Tre, and Andre, whose help have guided this book from its conception to its completion.

I thank my father and mother, Lee and Mildred Talley, for giving me life and constant inspiration.

I thank my brothers, Lee Jr., Reginald, and John Talley, for listening to me long distance, and believing in me.

I thank my sister, Georgette Talley Moss, for sharing my dream.

I thank my visible angel, Pat Iverson, for always encouraging and protecting me. Thank you for working on the logo.

I thank Monica Crayton, my prayer partner, for constant prayer and support.

I thank Avis Lamb Brown for motivation, advice, and for constantly asking me about the plan.

I thank Lynn James, Pam Lloyd, and Tangelar Sanders, my devoted readers, for being helpful from the beginning to the end of the book. Your votes of confidence always encouraged me.

I thank Fay Epps for all of our interesting conversations. I really appreciate all of your brilliant ideas.

I thank Defae Weaver of Precision Type, for helping to make my dream a reality.

I thank Johnny Iverson for helping me during a difficult time with my computer.

I thank Michele Henry, for giving me feedback, and love editing.

And last but not least, I would like to thank, Beverly Cannon, Pamela Whitehead, Linda Offord, Linda Sims, Veda Iverson, Reida and Freida Simmons, Lindell Crosby, Patricia Carroll, Juanita Pace, Bob Stoker, Bernice Sanders, Gwen Pearson, Raymond Owens, Rocky Taylor, Tanisha Price, Robin Franklin, Denise Foxx, Marilyn Hayes, Victoria Brown, James Brown, Linnie Simmons, Otherine Smith, Lillian Picket-Smith, Brenda Wilson, Bridgit Mosley, Lawanna Sherman, and Helen Williams for supporting and encouraging me every step of the way.

TABLE OF CONTENTS

Introduction		9
Chapter One	Black Hair Types	13
Chapter Two	Shampooing & Conditioning	19
Chapter Three	Hair Product Junkie	31
Chapter Four	Home Maintenance Guide	35
Chapter Five	Hair Cutting	49
Chapter Six	Hair Weaves & Extensions	59
Chapter Seven	Chemical Hair Relaxing	71
Chapter Eight	Hair Coloring	81
Chapter Nine	How to Select a Hairstylist	89
Chapter Ten	Frequently Asked Questions & Answers	95
Conclusion		107

Introduction

Black hair care has come a long way. I thank God we have more hair care options today. Do you remember how we use to almost pull our hair out of our scalps by braiding it so tightly we found it difficult to blink an eye? Do you remember how we use to single press, double press, and even pull press our curly hair only to have it quickly revert to its natural state? Do you remember the harsh chemical relaxers that caused our scalps to receive first and second degree burns? And oh yes, let us please not forget that dreadful, over-processed, drippy, hooked on plastic cap, jheri curl.

Today our hair care options are more advanced than ever. On the threshold of a new century, we are fortunate to have beauty treatments available that make our hair types more versatile when it comes to styling. Now, I am not recommending that you try everything that comes along. I am simply suggesting that you become aware of your best hair care options. With the assistance of your cosmetologist, you will be able to make the correct choices for you. Even though your look should reflect you, it should also be a team effort. Always consult your hairstylist so that he or she will be able to recommend a coiffure that will be suitable for your hair type, flatter your face, compliment your wardrobe, and accommodate your lifestyle.

Now, let me tell you about myself. For as long as I can remember, hair has fascinated me, and even though I've been in the beauty industry for over twenty years, I am still captivated. In my twenties, I attended Beauty College, and became a cosmetologist. The owner of the school recommended that I become an instructor because she felt that I demonstrated a strong desire to help people. After graduating from Beauty College I was hired by a major chemical relaxer manufacturer. While working in the test salon of that company I made some startling discoveries, and I will share this information with you throughout the book. A few years later, I was blessed to receive a scholarship to train as a cosmetology instructor. During my first year of teaching I was awarded "The Rookie of the Year" from the owner of the college. Receiving this award was very rewarding to me because that company owned thirty-two Beauty Colleges in the Texas-Oklahoma area. Years later that same company promoted me to Manager of Education of their largest Beauty College. This position allowed me the opportunity to manage, to teach, and to write beauty school curriculums. While teaching Beauty College, I worked part-time in several prestigious hair salons in Dallas. I have managed my own hair salon and gift store in a quaint shopping mall in the Dallas area for the last seven years. I absolutely love my work. Words cannot express how rewarding it is to make someone look and feel better because of a beauty service I gave. Well that's enough about me. I don't want you to think that I am trying to impress you with my credentials. (Yeah! Right!) Well, anyway, let us get to the reason you are reading this book.

Now, if you have thumbed through the pages of this book already, you will have noticed that I did not fill it with more hair pictures than hair information. If you wanted to see hairstyles, you could have easily purchased a hair magazine. Most hair books on the market today are filled with glossy pictures taken by a professional photographer of models dressed by professional fashion stylists. It is my opinion that those books do not contain enough useful information about Black hair care. I took the majority of the photographs in this book. I want you to know that all of the ladies in the photographs are probably just like you, ordinary, professional, Black women, but they are pretty special people to me. You see, they are my hair clients. I decided to use my hair clients instead of models because I wanted to keep this book real. After all, I wrote it to help you, today's Black woman.

Healthy Hair Care Tips For Today's Black Woman

Cheryl Talley Moss

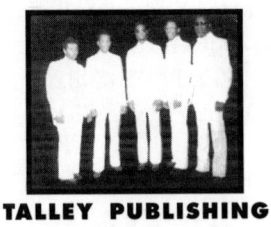

TALLEY PUBLISHING

COPYRIGHT © 1999 by Cheryl Talley Moss
All rights reserved.
Printed in the United States of America

No part of this book may be reproduced or transmitted in any form or by any means, electronic or mechanical, including photocopying, recording or by any information storage and retrieval systems, without the written permission from the publisher.

Library of Congress Catalog Card Number: 99-93781

ISBN: 0-9671491-0-X

Healthy Hair Care Tips for Today's Black Woman/Cheryl Talley Moss

Cover and layout design by Defae Weaver
Printing by Great Impressions
Photographs by Cheryl Talley Moss
Talley logo created by Bridget Mosley

Please send all permission requests to:

TALLEY PUBLISHING
c/o CHERYL TALLEY MOSS
P.O. BOX 870871
MESQUITE, TEXAS 75187-0871

FOR SHOWS OR APPEARANCES CALL
214-320-2300

CHAPTER ONE

BLACK HAIR TYPES

First of all, I want you to know that I wrote this chapter because I was tired of the misconceptions concerning Black hair. For so long Black women all over the world have been influenced to believe that our different hair types are difficult to style, to grow, and to maintain. For centuries we have been told that our hair is *bad.* Even today, the words *"good hair"* are used to describe any Black person's hair that is either straight or wavy. Some people consider curly and kinky hair types to be bad. Nothing could be further from the truth; *everyone can have good hair regardless of what type you may have.* **Good hair is simply hair that is healthy, attractively styled and manageable.** Now that I have gotten that off my chest, let me help you understand the composition of hair.

Hair is an extension of the skin and scalp. *Chemically speaking, all hair types are the same.* Everyone's hair (all races and nationalities) is mostly composed of a protein substance called keratin. *Physically speaking, all hair types are not the same.* In order to understand the differences, you must understand hair structure. Just like our skin, our hair has many layers. There are two major layers of hair, the cuticle and the cortex. I will be referring to these layers throughout the chapters of the book. *The outer layers of hair are called the cuticles.* **The more cuticle layers you have in a single strand of hair the more protection the hair has** against the elements, chemical processing, blow-drying, thermal curling, combing and brushing. **The curlier your natural hair is, the less cuticle layers you have**. *The cortex is the inner layer of the hair. This layer gives strength and elasticity to the hair.* Natural pigment (coloring) is contained in the cortex. Chemical relaxers, permanent waves and permanent hair coloring affect the cortex. The amount of hair layers (cuticle and cortex) will determine the diameter of your individual hair strand. This is called texture. Fine, medium and coarse are the three major hair textures. You can have a combination of all three textures on different parts of your head. By the way, **scalp hair grows about one half of an inch per month.** The growth of hair occurs more rapidly between the ages of twelve and thirty, but declines significantly between forty-five and sixty.

Many hairstylists try to put all Black hair into one category. My twenty years of experience in the beauty industry has allowed me to work with every hair type, and has taught me that this theory is not practical. There are several different Black hair types and each type is unique and different. Once you recognize the physical differences, you will be able to understand Black hair better. When you can identify your hair type, you will be able to make your hair (with the assistance of your hairstylist) the healthiest it can possibly be. And if you are a multi-cultural sister, you will learn how to properly care for your hair also.

Black hair can be straight, wavy, curly or kinky and it is not unusual for a person to have a combination of two or more types. When determining your hair type, look at an inch of virgin hair closest to your scalp. Virgin hair is natural hair that hasn't been processed with chemicals. So if your hair is chemically relaxed, examine your "new growth."

STRAIGHT HAIR

Straight hair has no curl or wave to it. *Contrary to popular belief, Black women can have straight hair.* Straight hair has more cuticle layers than any other type and it is very resistant to chemical services. This type of hair usually has an incredible shine because the cuticle layers lie flat and allow light to bounce off of its smooth surface easier than an uneven surface. Straight hair is also resistant to thermal curling. A soft body wave can give this hair type manageability and control.

Wavy Hair

Wavy hair has a definite "S" pattern to the hair shaft, and it tends to lay close to the scalp. This hair type is usually shiny. The cuticles lie almost flat giving the hair some shine, but not as much shine as straight hair. *Wavy hair also has a tendency to be frizzy.* Black women with this hair type can roller set or thermal curl the hair for a smoother look. Just remember that this hair type will revert to its original wavy state in humid conditions.

Curly Hair

Curly hair has a definite loop "S" pattern. It is usually very soft. Curly hair is not as shiny as straight or wavy hair because the cuticles do not lie flat. Today's Black women have more acceptance of their curly hair textures. I think that naturally curly hair looks absolutely fabulous (especially if it is cut short). Curly hair can also be chemically relaxed or thermal straightened to achieve the smoother styles that are popular today.

Kinky Hair

Kinky hair is very similar to curly hair. It is just more tightly curled. This hair type is usually extremely soft and dry. *Kinky hair will break off easily when combed*; however, you can grow kinky hair long into dreadlocks because you do not comb the hair. Most people think kinky hair is strong because of its tough appearance. Sometimes looks can be deceiving. *Kinky hair has the least amounts of cuticle layers, which means it is the weakest hair type.* Chemically relaxing this hair type can make it more manageable, but it will leave the hair in a weaker condition. Kinky hair has a dull appearance because light does not reflect off the cuticles because they do not lie flat. If you have this hair type, don't be discouraged because I am going to tell you how to make your hair stronger and healthier.

Have you determined your hair type yet? I am sure most of you knew already. Just remember you need at least an inch of virgin hair to be able to identify your hair type.

NOTES

CHAPTER TWO

Shampooing & Conditioning

Most Black women, over twenty years old, were taught as children to believe that we only needed to shampoo our hair once every two weeks. We were taught that shampooing too often would dry our hair out. In defense of our mothers, I must say that "back in the day," they used harsher shampoos that would leave our hair in a hard, brittle condition. Because those old shampoos would strip the hair of moisture, our mother's doing what they thought was best, would oil our scalps with heavy grease. You see, their mothers taught them that the grease would condition the hair. Believe it or not, some sisters still practice this "old school" hair regimen. For those of you that are still doing this, please, please stop!! *Grease cannot condition your hair and it will clog up your hair follicles.* (Don't worry about it. I will explain it to you very soon.)

SHAMPOOING

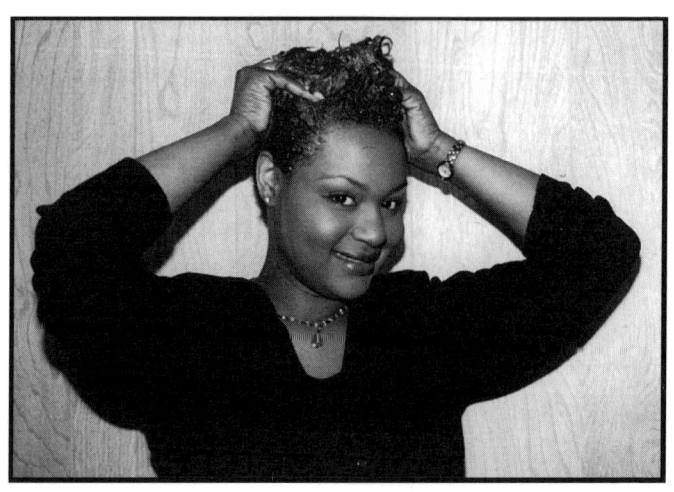

Today, shampoos are formulated for specific needs. *Most Black hair types are usually dry.* So, *select a moisturizing shampoo for dry or chemically treated hair.* Ask your stylist to recommend a shampoo for you or *look for shampoos that contain keratin, hydrolyzed vegetable protein, panthenol, and aloe vera.* Shampoos that contain some or all of these ingredients will deposit emollients in the hair that condition as the shampoo cleans. Make sure these ingredients are listed first on the shampoo bottle because the largest amount of an ingredient contained in a product is listed first.

Shampooing your hair will deposit moisture as well as remove dirt, oil, debris and styling products that can clog up the hair follicles (hair follicles are the pockets in the scalp that hold the hair root). Rinse the hair thoroughly to remove the shampoo scum. When you shower, you wouldn't want the soap scum to remain on your skin, would you? Leaving shampoo scum on your hair will defeat the purpose for shampooing it in the first place, and it can damage your hair. Be sure to use lukewarm water because hot water dries your hair out.

It is safe to shampoo all "virgin" hair types (hair that hasn't been chemically processed) daily. By the way, you can rinse or shampoo dreadlocks and braids in the shower once a day. Chemically relaxed hair must be shampooed (at least) once a week.

Dandruff

I think most dandruff shampoos are a waste of money. Let me explain to you why I feel this way. The top layer of the scalp continually sheds and is replaced. When these small, white scales on the scalp fall off freely, it is called **dry scalp**. Sometimes the flakes do not fall off and will accumulate on the scalp, this is called dandruff. The two types of dandruff are dry and greasy. **Dry dandruff** usually causes the scalp to itch. The major causes of this type of dandruff are:

- Poor circulation to the scalp,
- uncleanness,
- improper diet, and
- stress.

My experience has taught me that if the hair is shampooed at least once a week with a moisturizing shampoo, mild cases of dry dandruff usually will go away. During the shampoo the scalp is stimulated, blood circulation is increased, and the loose scales are washed away. **Greasy dandruff** will also make your scalp itch and can be very serious. The greasy, yellowish scales are a combination of dead skin and sebum. (Sebum is your natural scalp oil that is produced by the sebaceous glands.) Over the counter, medicated shampoos will help with light cases of greasy dandruff; however, if you have **seborrhea**, a heavy accumulation of greasy dandruff, where bleeding occurs, seek medical attention immediately. This condition can lead to permanent hair loss. Because bacteria is present in this scalp disorder, dandruff is contagious. All combs, brushes, and any other hair implements should not be shared with anyone.

Ringworm

Ringworm (Tinea) is a fungus that can appear on the scalp and skin. The small white or red patches are highly contagious and can lead to hair loss. This disease requires immediate medical attention. Ringworm is caused by vegetable parasites.

Sisters please remember this: Experts agree that you must keep your scalp clean in order to resist scalp disorders. So, throw out the myth that we only need to shampoo our hair once every two weeks. **To maintain healthy hair, be sure to shampoo all hair types at least once a week** and always follow your shampoo with a good...

Conditioning

Because most Black hair types tend to be dry, you should follow every shampoo with a **moisturizing conditioner**. *Look for conditioners that contain protein, keratin, panthenol, lanolin, and vitamin E.* Conditioners with these ingredients will help to make your hair stronger, restore moisture, and assist in preventing future damage. You see, just about everything we do to our hair can damage it. Apply the conditioner to clean, towel-dried hair and leave it on between fifteen and thirty minutes. Be sure to concentrate on the hair ends the most. Cover the hair with a plastic cap or an electric heating cap to increase the conditioner's benefits.

Conditioners cannot permanently repair severely damaged hair, but they will help to prevent your hair from getting any worse. Conditioners protect the hair from being defenseless against everyday styling, curling irons, chemical services, and even air. Yes, I said air! Think about it, everything that is exposed to air dries out. Food dries out, water evaporates, your skin (if exposed to the air for long periods of time without protection) will dry out. Why should your hair be any different?

Don't neglect your hair if you are wearing dreadlocks or braids. Always use a moisturizing conditioner weekly. By the way, dreadlocks should be given a hot oil treatment every two weeks to make them softer. Use natural oils (like lavender, jojoba, and rosemary) and be sure to apply the oil between the hair partings. Lubricating your dreads with hot oil will prevent them from breaking off. This is a common problem for people that wear dreads. Now let's talk about the benefits of a hot oil treatment because (according to my research) many sisters are confused about what it will actually do. Oil is a lubricant, and will help to make your hair softer. But oil is not moisture. It is true that we need to replenish the oil our hair loses (especially during chemical relaxing). That is why oil is contained in most moisturizing conditioners; however, this does not mean that you should skip your weekly moisturizing conditioner treatments.

Chemically relaxed hair is usually the driest hair type, and it can break off easily at the ends (if the hair isn't conditioned regularly). In order for it to remain healthy, all chemically relaxed hair must receive a penetrating moisturizing conditioner at least once a week to counteract the drying that occurs from the relaxer applications. *Penetrating moisturizing conditioners are generally thick in consistency and will help to restore the moisture balance in the hair.*

A **moisturizing reconstructive conditioner** should be given at least once a month. (The week after the chemical relaxer application would be best.) *If your hair is double-processed* (with a chemical relaxer and permanent hair color) *use a moisturizing reconstructive conditioner every week.* Reconstructive conditioners are generally thinner in consistency, and will restore moisture and stability to the hair by penetrating into the cortex layer. They will also improve hair texture, increase elasticity, and equalize porosity. (Porosity is the ability of the hair to absorb moisture.) If you fail to condition your hair at least once a week, your ends will break off as fast as your hair will grow out. This **break-n-grow pattern** is what has convinced many sisters that our hair cannot grow out to long lengths.

If our hair is cared for properly it can grow out to long lengths (even if it is chemically relaxed). You see, my experience working in the test salon of a major chemical relaxer manufacturer taught me that when the hair is chemically relaxed to a smooth straight texture it loses about fifty percent of its original strength when wet and about twenty-five percent when in a dry state. Because of this loss of strength (especially when wet) you have to make sure that you put back into the hair the protein and the moisture the relaxer took out by conditioning it regularly.

Just for the record, let me say that *I do not like homemade conditioners.* Be careful about using homemade remedies (like mixtures of mayonnaise and garden vegetables) as conditioners. Conditioners and shampoos are now formulated with organic ingredients. *Homemade remedies are not as effective and can be more costly than hair conditioners that are specifically designed for your hair type.* **By the way, don't waste your money buying cheap hair products because you will end up spending more money in the long run.** You will have to buy cheaper hair products more often because generic brands are usually watered down. I truly believe you get what you pay for.

One more thing… *I don't recommend anyone substituting a leave-in conditioner for a weekly moisturizing conditioner.* They do not penetrate into the hair shaft, and contain fillers (oil, wax and balsam) that coat the hair shaft. I consider leave-in conditioners to be a temporary fix to a hair problem. They should be used in emergency situations only. They will not make the hair stronger, but they will help to make the hair feel softer; however, excessive use of leave-in conditioners can weigh the hair down leaving it limp and flat.

Now, let me tell you about Monica, a regular client of mine. She used to have dry, brittle, damaged hair with split ends. Monica, a working wife and mother, has a very busy schedule. She felt it was only necessary to have her hair shampooed and conditioned once every two weeks. Because her hair was breaking off excessively, I recommended that she come into the salon once a week for a conditioning treatment until I could stop her hair from breaking off. You see, I knew Monica's hair was starving for moisture. After about three months, I told Monica that I could not continue to do her hair because I knew her hair would not stop breaking off until she could commit to having her hair shampooed and conditioned once a week by me or herself. I also told her that I felt uncomfortable about taking her money knowing her hair would never improve. Monica said that she appreciated my honesty and to make a long story short, she began to take time out of her busy schedule for herself. She made weekly visits to the salon. After about four weeks, her hair started to improve tremendously. Take a look at Monica's beautiful, long, healthy hair. I'm sure you've heard of the old saying, "seeing is believing." Monica may not be a famous celebrity, but her hair sure makes her look like one.

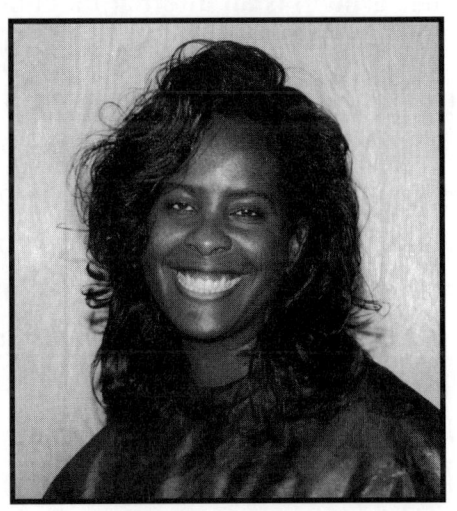

I know everyone cannot afford (or has the time for) weekly salon visits. Just try to shampoo and condition your hair at least once a week because your hair must be nourished to remain healthy.

Now, *there are many hair conditioners on the market that claim to promote hair growth. They will not.* Note: Doctors can prescribe drugs to help with hair loss. I am not including physician-prescribed medications or over-the-counter products that slow hair loss or promote hair growth (like Rogaine®) in this category. *I am referring to the products sold through tiny ads placed in the back of magazines.* I'm sure you have seen the ads with the picture of the woman with thick, artificial looking hair hanging down to her ankles. Don't be fooled or tricked into purchasing conditioners that claim to make your hair grow unrealistically long. The simple truth is . . . **hair growth is an internal function of the body**. There are no wonder conditioners or miracle pills that can make your hair grow faster. Eating a balanced diet, drinking plenty of water, exercising (aerobically) at least four days a week, taking multi-vitamins, getting the proper amount of rest, and keeping your life as stress-free as possible are the best things you can do to make your body, mind, and hair the healthiest it can be. So called "**magic products**" that do not have scientific clinical studies to support them **will not speed up hair growth**, and they are usually strategically marketed to Black women. So please, please do not waste your money buying any of them. *Always consult your doc-*

tor or hairstylist before purchasing any hair product that promises to do unrealistic things. Spending the money you worked hard to earn on products that claim to produce supernatural results is a sure way of turning yourself into a "hair product junkie." Now if you don't know what a "hair product junkie" is... well, just read the next chapter. (It's only a few pages.) I sincerely hope you aren't *one*.

NOTES

CHAPTER THREE

Hair Product Junkie

Every time I hear or see a new **"miracle product"** advertised, I just want to scream. I don't know how the inventors of this junk and the executives that market it can sleep at night. They prey upon the vulnerabilities of innocent people offering false hope to those with hair problems.

Every year, my sisters spend billions of hard earned dollars on hair products that will not do what they claim to do. A few years ago, the manufacturers of a popular, shampoo and conditioner claimed to make your hair as strong as horse hair. The company made millions of dollars, and the products made your hair as hard as a brick. People were convinced that their hair was healthier until it began to break off.

Do you remember the infomercial that advertised a product that claimed to make curly hair straight "naturally?" The manufacturers of that product sold it to sisters all over the world. They claimed the product was not a chemical and that it was safe to apply over hair that was chemically relaxed. Well, you know the end of the story. Most sisters that used it lost the majority of their hair, and some women went bald. The company quickly went out of business, and is still involved in lawsuits. A few of my clients left me for a short while because they fell for the hype. I welcomed them back with open arms, like a mother does for her children that stray away. But there wasn't much I could do for any of them because that product left their hair in a terrible breaking-off condition. I had to cut the damaged hair off so that they could start over and grow it out.

If a hair product sounds too good to be true, it is. Please take my advice: **Don't purchase "quick fixes" and products that claim to give unbelievable results**. Trust me, other "miracle products" will come along soon. Have you heard about the latest one? I will call it *instant damage repair*. What a joke, this product claims to repair any hair damage, instantly. Please do not fall for it because if you do, you will find yourself falling for anything and everything that comes along. Do not let any one turn you into a "hair product junkie."

"**Hair Product Junkie's**" will shop at beauty supply stores, supermarkets, and discount stores; anywhere they can . . . looking for the latest hair gimmick to purchase. Women come into my salon almost everyday seeking the "miracle solution" to their hair problems. Women with thin, fine hair keep asking me about thickening shampoos. I have tried many of them. Let me just say, they cannot and will not thicken your hair. Shampoos cannot permanently change your hair texture. I do not care how expensive they may be. Thickening shampoos will leave a little coating on your hair shaft, and will give you a little more lift. (But you can slightly increase your hair diameter by using a small amount of styling gel on your hair.) Ask your hairstylist to recommend the appropriate products for your hair type. Most salons retail the same styling products their stylists use. I am not going to endorse any product lines, but I will tell you which hair products you should avoid using. Do not use hair products that contain alcohol, (with the exception of a dry holding hair spray). Avoid using super holding gels and finishing spritz. Excessive use of super holding gels will rob your hair of its moisture and will help to create uncontrollable flakes. Frequent use of finishing spritz will make your hair hard and hard hair will easily break off. **Do not thermal curl your hair using finishing spritz.** Most spritz contain acrylic (the same ingredient in sculpture nail products) that should not be baked into your hair. If you look on the back of any spritz bottle, you will see "**Caution: Flammable. Do not use near open flame or while smoking**." Why you or any hairstylist would use spritz in conjunction with a hot curling iron bewilders me. Styling spritz is a finishing product designed to maintain hard hair styles. It should only be used after the hairstyle is created. While I am on the subject, let me just say that **wearing hard "patent leather looking" hairstyles all of the time will quickly lead to unhealthy hair.** Please remember that it is impossible to have healthy hair if you are constantly drying it out. To keep hair healthy between salon visits, you need a daily home maintenance guide.

CHAPTER FOUR

HOME MAINTENANCE GUIDE

You walk out of the hair salon looking good and feeling like a million bucks with your beautiful new hairstyle! You get home and you say to yourself… Now what do I need to do to maintain my "do?" Has this ever happened to you? Did you see the movie, *Friday*? Do you remember the scene where Regina King's character sits upright in her bed all night long trying to maintain her hairstyle? That scene is hysterically funny because we can all relate to it, but in real life we would get neck cramps attempting to sleep like that. Let me show you how you can get some restful sleep and still maintain your hairstyle.

If you are wearing a smooth or straight hairstyle, *wrap your hair at night with a silk or satin scarf* to maintain your style, to retain moisture, and to reduce stress to the hair. *Do not use a cotton scarf, because cotton absorbs moisture and will make your hair dry out.*

If you need to roll your hair at night, always wear smooth, plastic rollers. *Do not use sponge rollers*, because this type of roller will pull your hair out. Some people wrap tissue around sponge rollers before using them, but your hair will still catch on the plastic part of the roller. And please, please, please, **don't sleep in velcro rollers** because your hair will break off as you toss and turn during the night. If you don't believe me, take a look at the velcro rollers of any one that uses them. They are generally covered with hair. Always wear a satin hair bonnet to retain moisture, to keep your rollers in place, and to prevent you from adding stress to your hair.

If you like to wear your hair in a curlier style and find it uncomfortable to sleep in rollers, try pin curling your hair at

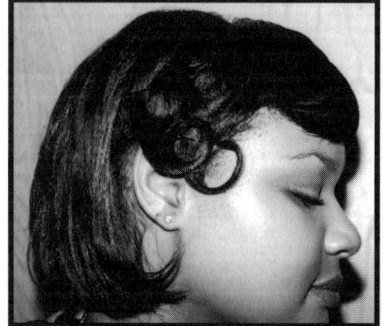

night. *Pin curls are easy to sleep in, and they will not stress your hair.* Comb smooth a small section of hair. Starting at the ends, wind your hair around and around until you reach the scalp. Secure the pin curl by inserting a bobby pin through the center. The size of your pin curls will determine the size of your curls. In other words, the smaller your pin curls are, the tighter your curls will be (and vise versa). If you try this technique on wet hair, be sure to use smooth pin curl clips. Placing bobby pins in wet pin curls will leave indentation marks in your hair after it dries.

Now, for those of you that are addicted to thermal curling your hair everyday, I need to let you know that **I do not recommend using a curling iron to touch up your hairstyle between salon visits.** The heat from the curling iron will degrade the hair and cause it to break off. In humid conditions, hair that has been damaged by excessive thermal curling will look dry and frizzy. If you are one of those women that curl your hair everyday, please, please stop!! Your hair will not be able to endure this type of treatment for long because **every time you thermal curl your hair, you break down a cuticle layer.** Lets face it, the reason you thermal curl your hair every day is because you *have* to curl it every day. Your hair is damaged, and it will not look smooth unless you press the cuticles flat with a curling iron. And before the day is over, you are right back where you started (with frizzy hair). Am I right? I know I'm right! You see you are not alone, I use to fry my hair daily too! For those of you that insist on burning your ears and frying your hair daily, please, please try to at least use a moisturizing cream to act as a buffer for your hair. Be sure to remember that if you thermal curl your hair between salon visits you will be baking whatever is on your hair (dirt, debris, and styling products) into your hair. Try a roller set for a change because you can achieve the same results, and a roller set will last longer.

Because Black women generally do not produce oil on our scalps as quickly as Caucasian women, and due to the fact that the majority of Black women wear a chemical relaxer that tends to dry our scalps out even more, it is okay to occasionally use a light oil on our scalps. A light oil will not clog your hair follicles, but heavy grease certainly will. Please do not forget what I said about "miracle products." All of those magic greases you tried in the past didn't work. Come on now admit it, 'cause y'all know you bought some! Hair growth starts from within your body. **Grease does not promote hair growth**.

If you have to shampoo and style your hair between regular salon visits, I recommend that you use the following hair products because they are light and non-drying. **Be sure to ask your hairstylist to recommend a brand name for you.**

Home Maintenance Hair Products

1. A gentle **shampoo**, to clean and moisturize the hair (formulated for dry or chemically relaxed hair);
2. A **conditioner**, to protect the hair, and to restore moisture and protein balance;

3. A **setting lotion**, to create body, and to give sheen;
4. A light **styling gel**, to keep tapered sides and nape areas smooth (optional);
5. An **oil sheen spray**, to add gloss and to lusterize the hair (can be used on all hair types);
6. A dry **holding hair spray**, to hold the hair in place, and to prevent hairstyles from drooping and frizzing in humid conditions. Be sure to use sparingly. All dry hair sprays contain a form of mild alcohol (usually SDA 40);
7. A very **light oil**, to loosen roller sets, can be used as a light scalp oil, and to be used as a hot oil treatment for dreadlocks and braids;
8. A **moisturizing cream**, to use as a leave-in moisturizer for extremely dry hair, and to act as a curling iron buffer.

As we head toward the new millennium, one of the most recycled hairstyling techniques out is the versatile roller set. Not since the 1970s when the weekly roller set was the way to get your "do" has roller sets been this popular. Today's Black women want a hairstyle that is going to last, but they don't want to wear hard hairstyles because **wearing hard hair can be very drying**. A roller set is a hairstyling technique that will allow women with chemically relaxed hair to change their straight hair texture (temporarily) into hairstyles that are curlier or have more volume and body. *A roller set will last about a week, and is also the perfect hairstyle for women that exercise and perspire from their scalp.* Before you workout, comb your hair into a ponytail. Secure it loosely

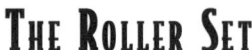

with a terry cloth ponytail band. Be sure to wear a sweatband around your hairline while you exercise. After your workout, blow-dry your hair at the scalp area on a cool setting. Take your ponytail down, comb it out and go.

THE ROLLER SET

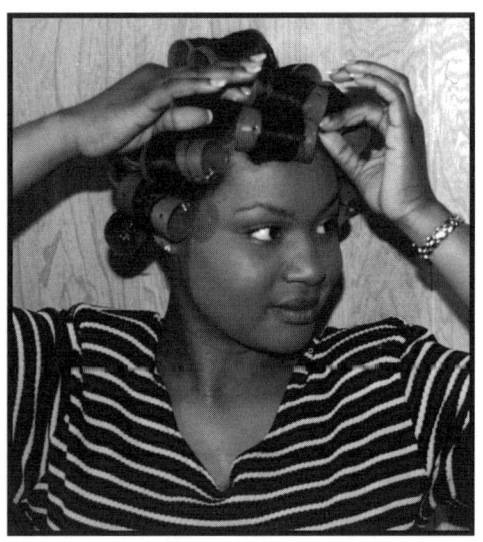

One of the least damaging hairstyles you can do at home is a roller set. For smooth results, follow this procedure:

- ❖ Shampoo and condition your hair.
- ❖ Apply setting lotion to towel-dried hair. The setting lotion will give the hair more body and control.
- ❖ Using a wide tooth comb, start at the ends of the hair, gently comb the hair working toward the scalp to remove tangles. Take small sections and comb your hair smooth. Be sure to comb your hair gently, this is

very important, because the hair is weak (and will break easily) when it is wet.
- ❖ Always use smooth magnetic rollers. The larger the roller, the larger the curl will be (and vise versa). Starting at the top of your head, section off a piece of hair that is the same diameter and length of your roller.
- ❖ Comb this section of hair smooth, and beginning at the hair ends, wrap the hair around the roller. Keep rolling the hair around the roller until it reaches the scalp.
- ❖ Secure the roller in place with a roller clamp or a roller clip.
- ❖ Dry your hair under a hooded hair dryer. Be sure to let the hair dry completely because if you don't your hair will frizz. The drying time can be anywhere from one-half hour to two hours (depending on your hair length).

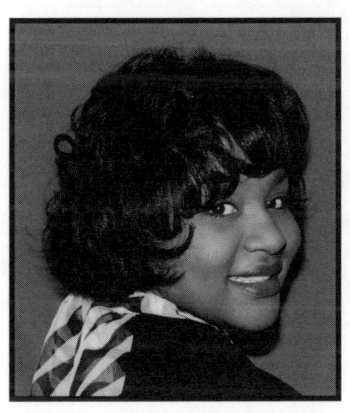 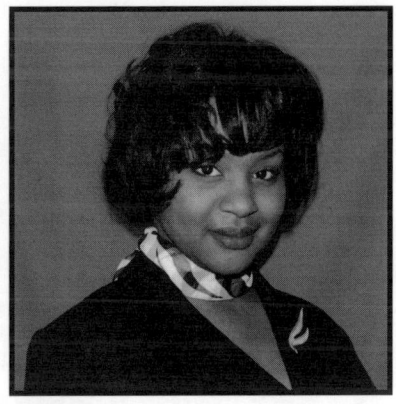

Try a roller set for soft, silky, fabulous looking hair. Alisa's gorgeous hairstyle will last about a week.

Cheryl Talley Moss

THE WRAPP

We are entering an era in which sisters want styling versatility. The wrapp is a quick way to achieve a smooth style with incredible body. Your head acts as one gigantic roller. For incredible results, follow this quick and simple procedure:

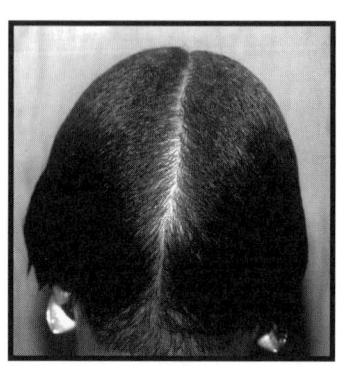
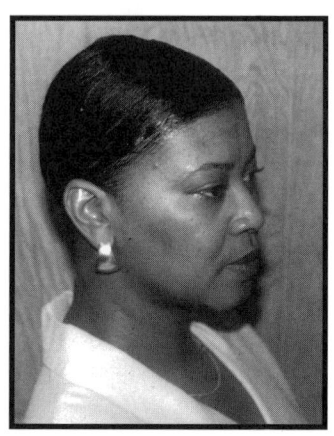

- ❖ Apply setting lotion to clean, towel-dried hair.
- ❖ Gently comb your hair smooth.
- ❖ Part your hair down the center from the front to the back of your head.
- ❖ Comb the top right and back section flat around your head and into the left section. Comb the left back and left top section around your head, into the right section (keeping the hair smooth as you go).
- ❖ Apply a small amount of a light styling gel on the hair ends to keep your hair in place.
- ❖ Dry your hair under a hooded hair dryer. Your hair can take anywhere from one to two hours to dry.

Do not put any type of hairpins into the wrapp while your hair is wet. If you do, you will have crinkled hair when it dries. And please, please *do not brush wet hair into a wrapp* (or any other hairstyle), *unless you want to instantly thin your hair out.* You must never forget that chemically relaxed hair is weaker when wet.

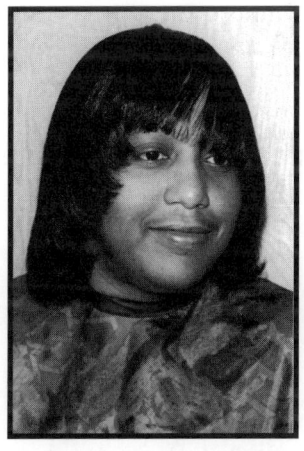

The wrapp allows Pamela to get this sleek effect. Her medium to long length tresses spill forward with incredible body.

Cheryl's wrapp was thermal curled in the crown area to give a more dramatic effect.
Alisa Moss, stylist.
Photo by Andre Moss.

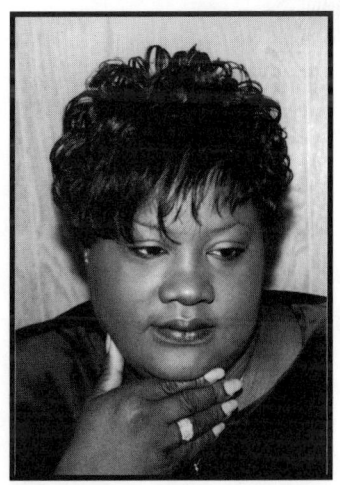

Cheryl Talley Moss

BLOW-DRYING

I do not recommend blow-drying any hair type that has been chemically relaxed. Always remember that **pulling on hair when it is in its weakest state will really damage it**. For those of you that insist on blow-drying your hair and making it lose some of its elasticity, each time you do it, I recommend that you pre-dry your hair under a hooded hair dryer. If you are still using one of those old fashioned pick or brush blow-dryer attachments on chemically relaxed hair, please, please, stop! You are ripping your hair out! Throw those ancient attachments away! The pick attachment was originally designed to blow-out an "Afro" on curly or kinky hair types. I attended one of the largest hairstyling shows and was appalled to see a platform hairstyling artist still using a pick blow-dryer attachment. Because I was sitting only a few yards from the stage, and due to the sophisticated lighting system, I could see the models chemically relaxed hair break off each time the hairstylist yanked the pick attachment through her wet hair. For those of you that are addicted to using a blow-drying attachment (on chemically relaxed hair) do not continue to abuse your hair this way, and you certainly should not pay a professional hairstylist to rip your hair out.

It is okay to blow-dry straight or wavy hair types, and it is a very simple procedure. To save on blow-drying time, make sure your shampooed and conditioned hair is thoroughly towel-dried.

- ❖ Starting at the scalp, using a plastic vent brush with plastic bristles, gently lift the hair closest to your scalp and blow-dry it.
- ❖ Make sure you dry all of the hair at the scalp area first.
- ❖ Next, dry the middle part of your hair strands.
- ❖ Finally, dry your hair ends.

Most women make the mistake of blow-drying their hair ends first. **You need to always dry your hair ends last because your ends are the oldest part of your hair and will be the driest and the most fragile.**

THERMAL CURLING

I do not recommend using electric rollers on chemically relaxed hair. Most women abuse their hair by leaving the hot rollers in the hair longer than necessary. Many women will leave the hot rollers in their hair (between ten and fifteen minutes) while they apply their facial make-up. Leaving electric rollers in chemically relaxed hair longer than five minutes will remove moisture. So, unless your hair is naturally straight or wavy, I wouldn't even go there.

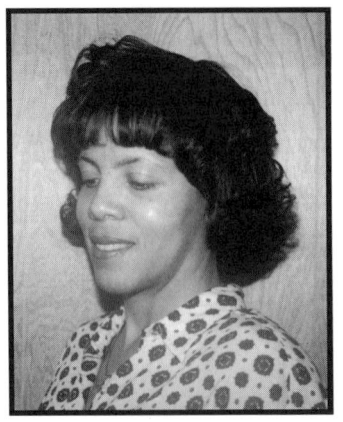

This modern version of the "Flip" was achieved by thermal curling the hair. Denise is an active "no-fuss" kind of a woman. She loves a hair "do" that is low maintenance.

Pam's tresses were thermal curled in the same direction of the wrapp to create this stunning look.

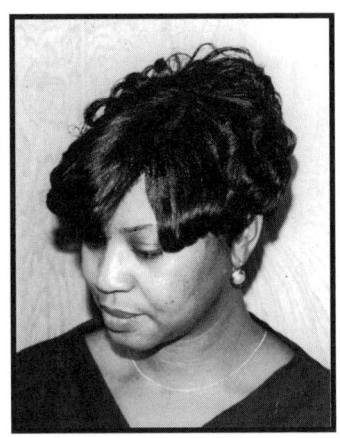

If you need to thermal curl your hair, use the inexpensive electric curling irons that allow you to set the temperature to low, medium, or high. Always *use the low or medium setting* (unless you have naturally straight or wavy hair). Never use professional Marcel curling irons because you will only end up burning your hair. This type of curling iron gets extremely hot. One wrong move can you give you a first or second-degree burn. A professional hairstylist is trained to manipulate the curling irons so that your hair is in the curling irons very briefly.

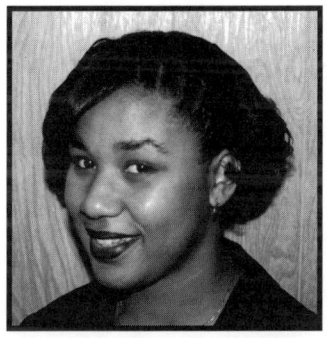

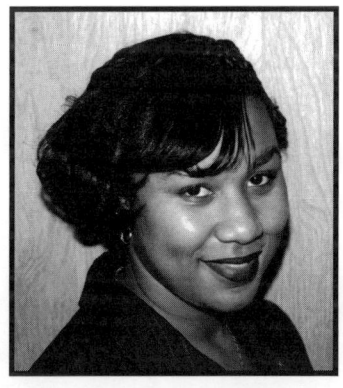

Two-strand twists were combined with soft thermal curls to give Veda this free flowing design.

Just like electric rollers, most women keep curling irons in their hair longer than necessary. The curling irons only need to be in your hair for a few seconds to curl it. I can look at a head of hair and will be able to tell if you frequently thermal curl your hair. So, if your hair is damaged, and your hairstylist asks you how often you curl your hair, don't lie, he or she probably already knows. **And please, remember, don't allow yourself to become addicted to thermal curling your hair everyday. This type of hair abuse will quickly make you need a serious haircut.**

NOTES

CHAPTER FIVE

Hair Cutting

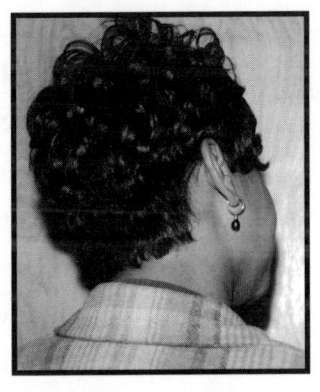

The foundation of every hairstyle is the haircut. Everything else that you do to your hair supports the cut. Hair coloring, chemical hair relaxing, and hair styling all work with the captain of the team, the haircut. A good haircut should compliment your facial features, hair texture, hair type, and body structure. Your lifestyle and the amount of time you desire to spend on styling your hair must also be considered. A good haircut will keep your coiffure's shape. I will not tell you how to cut your own hair because this is a service you need to leave to the professionals. *I do not recommend that anyone attempt to cut his or her own hair* (even if you are a hairstylist). How can you? You do not have eyes in the back of your head. You will only end up butchering your hair.

Please, please do not go to "chop shops" that specialize in quick, cheap haircuts because you will most likely end up with a mess. And honey, as far as your hair is concerned, there is nothing worse than a terrible haircut. "Fly in fly out" beauty shops train their hairstylists to cut hair fast. They do not concentrate on the quality of each individual haircut. Making sure the haircut is flattering to the client should be their main consideration. "Chop shops" have a habit of always forgetting that the client has a body beyond the shoulders.

To keep your hair healthy, you should have it trimmed every four to eight weeks. Having your hair trimmed regularly will prevent split ends. If split ends are not trimmed off consistently, they will continue to split up your hair shaft. In other words, you have to nip split hair ends in the bud. Think of it this way, hair with damaged split ends is just like an old bed sheet with a rip in it. If you do not mend the rip, it will continue to split. So, you see, **trimming your hair regularly is like preventative maintenance.**

Let me tell you about (I will call her) Elisa, a regular weekly client. Elisa wore a short haircut and chemical relaxer for about three years. Even though I always kept Elisa's haircut fresh and fashionable, she decided to grow her hair out for a completely new look. This was cool with me because I absolutely love to change my client's hair from time to time. It keeps them happy and excited about their personal appearance. So we developed a "hair growing out plan" for Elisa. Every six weeks she would receive a chemical relaxer retouch, and I would trim her hair ends. Every week she would receive a shampoo and conditioning treatment. It took us about twenty months to achieve healthy, shoulder length hair. Elisa was very proud of her long hair, so proud that she began to *trip*. Every time I tried to trim her split ends, she refused to allow me to snip off a centimeter of her hair. You see, she thought the way to maintain long hair was not to trim it. No matter how many times I explained to her that trimming the hair was not the same as cutting it, she refused to let me do it. I need to let you know that this all happened early in my career, during a period I allowed my clients to intimidate me. At the time, I thought I should not say anything to my clients that would make them stop coming to me. Well, after about a year of neglecting her split ends, Elisa's beautiful healthy tresses turned into knotted, split end messes. Because it was breaking off, she had to have her damaged hair cut off and ended up right back where she started with a short (but cute because I did it) haircut. Elisa and I learned an important lesson. That incident taught me how to be more professional. From that day on, I knew that I had to take control of my business. I told all of my clients what I really thought was best for their hair no matter how much I knew they disagreed with me. I was totally honest with them, and if that meant they would leave me to go to another hairstylist, then I would just have to adjust. Sometimes, you have to give it to them straight. It's like my momma always said, "You win some, you lose some."

Now, let me tell you about Reida and Freida, my teenage, identical twin clients. When they started coming to me, both of them had over-processed, damaged hair that was breaking off and in desperate need of a cut. I recommended that they both get short haircuts to remove the damaged hair. Reida did not want all of her 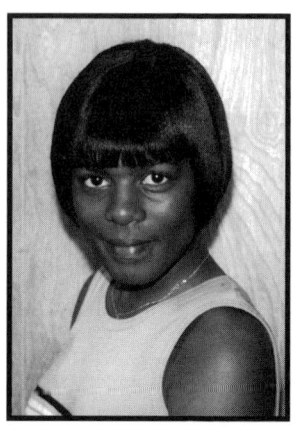 damaged hair cut off because she felt uncomfortable about having short hair. Freida, on the other hand, was excited about having her hair cut short. She told me that she had secretly yearned for a short haircut because she wanted to

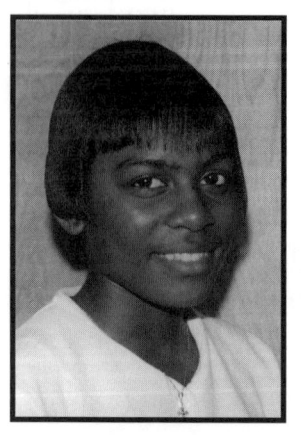 look a little different from her twin; furthermore, she had always admired short haircuts. As you can see, they are attractive girls with beautiful, oval face shapes that allow them to wear just about any type of haircut. So, I cut Reida's hair into a medium length bob (with the understanding that if I could not stop her hair from breaking

off, it had to go) and Freida's hair was cut into a short (two inch) layer. Because Reida's hair was not cut short enough to remove all of the damaged hair, it continued to break off; however, Freida stopped the break-n-grow process immediately. I eventually cut Reida's hair (just like her sister's original haircut) eight weeks later. Well, seeing *is* believing. Freida's hair (after six months) is longer. The point I am trying to make is this: It is impossible to hang on to damaged hair; it will break off anyway. Reida and Freida are young, and sometimes you have to prove things to young (sensitive) ladies. But I just do not understand why grown women try to hang on to "see-through" damaged hair. They ineffectively try to hide the damage by wearing glued down ponytails everyday. It doesn't make sense to hold on to damaged, lifeless hair because it will eventually break off anyway.

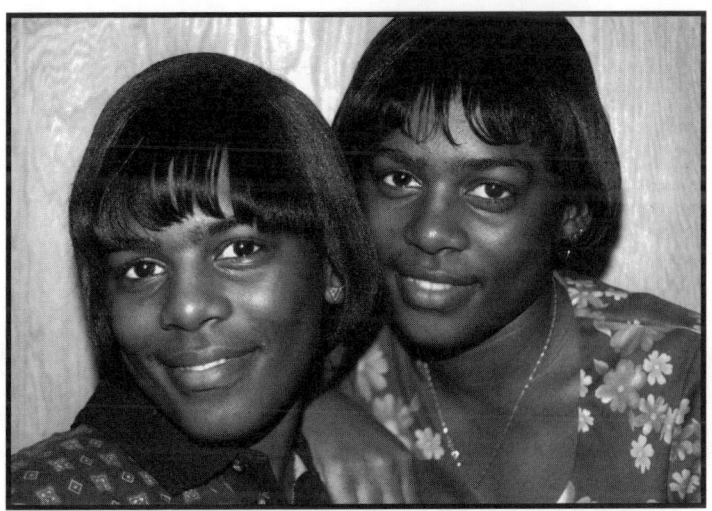

By the way, Reida now loves short hair, and Freida wants to grow her hair longer — that's teenagers for you!

As I said before, don't try to cut your own hair; however, here are some tips you need to consider. A good haircut should be very easy to style because it will quickly permit the hair to just fall into place. Do not take pictures of hairstyles to your stylist that are impossible to achieve on your hair. You would not believe how many women with thin, fine hair ask me to cut their hair just like Oprah's.

If you see a sister with a beautiful haircut, don't be afraid to ask her who cut her hair. My clients tell me that they are flattered when someone asks them who does their hair. Most hair clients cannot wait to tell people how great they think their hairstylist is. Any good hairstylist will tell you that the majority of their new clients are direct referrals from their regular clients.

If you are wearing your curly or kinky hair in a "natural" or an "Afro" you need a hairstylist that is trained to cut this hairstyle. It requires a unique hair cutting technique. I like to cut the "natural" when my client's hair is dry because your hair will stretch when it is wet and will contract (or shrink) when dry. So, to get the exact shape and length you want your hair to have, you should tell your hairstylist that you would prefer to have your hair cut dry. The "natural" is popular right now because everything that is old is new again and a lot of sisters are just tired of having their hair chemically relaxed. Most sisters that wear their hair in a "natural" have it cropped short. Short cuts are popular because busy women feel more comfortable with short hair. It is very easy to maintain and is more youthful looking. But before you go running off to the nearest beauty salon trying to take years off your age, I need to tell you that if you have your hair cut into any extremely short hairstyle, be sure you have the confidence to pull it off. **You have to have high self-esteem to be able to wear your hair very short**, it is a very revealing hairstyle and you will not have any hair to distract or camouflage your face.

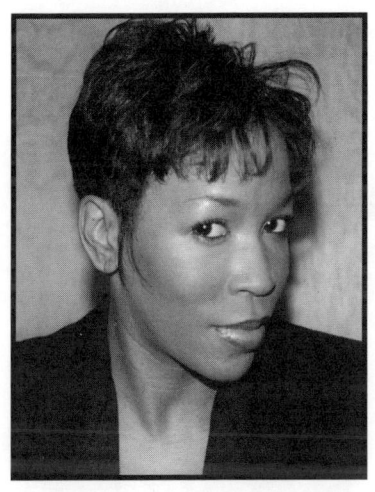

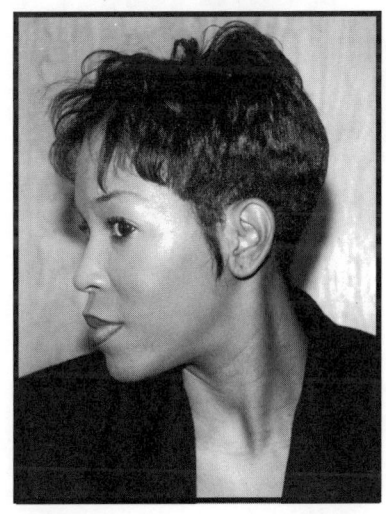

This isn't your average short bob. The precise cut features spiking through the top and is sure to gain attention anywhere Lynn goes.

For medium to long lengths of hair that is chemically relaxed, I recommend that you have your hairstylist cut your hair after the relaxer application. The natural curl pattern will be permanently straightened. Your hair in this state will allow your hairstylist to give you a precise haircut. If you wear your hair cut short and chemically relaxed, ask your hairstylist to cut your hair before the relaxer application. This will allow the hair to lay closer to the scalp for a smoother look.

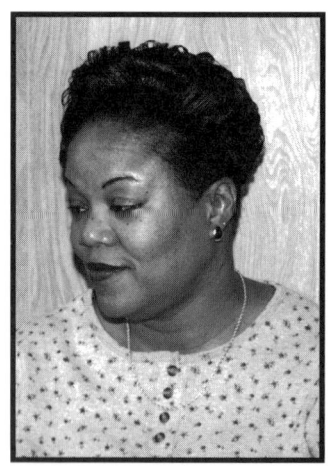

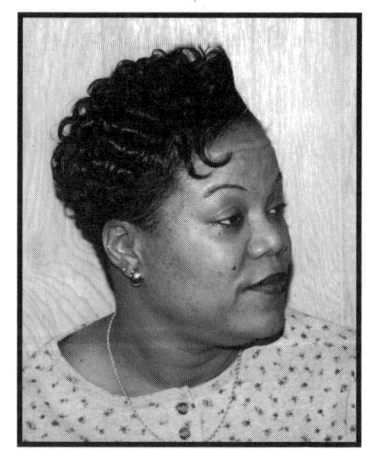

Avis took a styling leap by going ultra short! This head-hugging crop has sleek appeal at the sides and is absolutely maintenance free!

Thin hair will look fuller if it is layered or cut into one length. If you have very thick hair, don't have it cut extremely short if it is chemically relaxed because it will look like a porcupine when it isn't thermal curled.

The bob is the most popular haircut for chemically relaxed hair. There are many different variations of the bob. It is a very versatile haircut that has a classy look and it is easy to style and maintain at any hair length. Short bobs require having the hair layered and tapered at the neckline and temple areas. To prevent shorter bobs from looking like someone put a chili bowl on your head and chopped your hair off, you need to go to a stylist that is trained in precision hair cutting techniques.

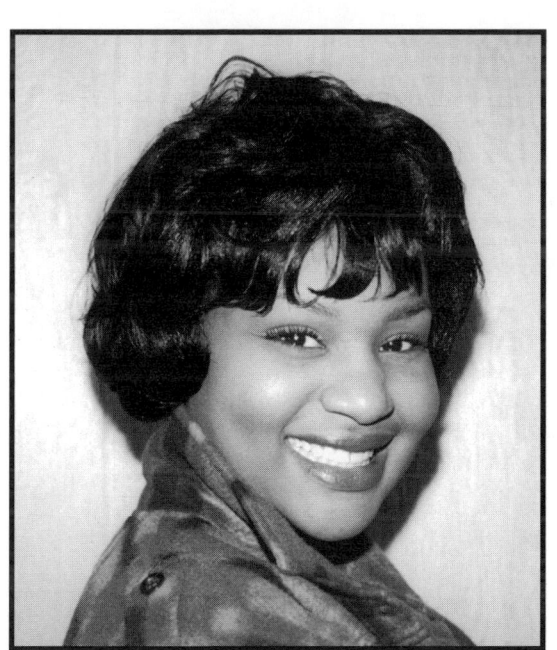

Alisa's conservative style doesn't have to be boring. Soft layers update this classic bob.

Every haircut should be versatile. Don't allow yourself to be locked into one hairstyle. So, in order to get a haircut that will allow you to create various styles, have your hair cut by a reputable hairstylist. Be sure to remember that routine trims every four to eight weeks will keep split ends away. **Don't be cheap when it comes to your haircut**! I said it before and I will say it again, you get what you pay for. And honey, the only thing you can do with a terrible haircut is add some glamour to it. Now, if you don't know what "added glamour" is, it's okay. Read on. I'll explain it to you in the next chapter.

CHAPTER SIX

HAIR WEAVES & EXTENSIONS

Most women, at one time or another, experiment with wigs, hairpieces, weaves, extensions or braids. I like to think of it as "added glamour." Some women put pieces into their hair to give it a fuller look, while others do it to give their hair some extra length or to cover bald and thinning spots. Other women add glamour to their natural hair because it is damaged. But the majority of women do it just because they want to change their look temporarily. Whatever your reason may be for adding a little glamour, there are some things you should consider.

There are many different ways to change your look. Think about how long you want to leave the "added glamour" in your hair. This will determine the method you choose. I recommend the following techniques for long-term hair extensions.

Long-Term Hair Extensions

Track Weave is my favorite method of long-term hair extensions. Your natural hair is braided into cornrows. Tracks of hair (hair stitched together on a weft) are sewn onto your cornrow braids. The sewn in tracks of hair will not fall out and you can move the weave any way you want it. Another long-term hair extension option is **Interlocking Braids**. Your hair is braided into small individual braids. As your hair is being braided, two or more inches (in width) of loose hair extensions are combined with your natural hair that is left out of the braid. **Micro Braids** is a hair extension technique that is also used for long-term. Micro braids are very similar to interlocking braids except they are braided from the scalp area to the hair ends and are much smaller. Another long-term technique is called **Extension Braids**. They are similar to micro braids except they are larger in size. **Hair Infusion** is another method of long-term hair extensions that was made famous by Janet Jackson. This method allows the greatest hair mobility. Strands of loose hair extensions are attached to your natural hair with a special glue. This method must be professionally attached and removed. All long-term hair extension methods cost between $400.00 and $800.00 for a full head. *Long-term hair extensions should not be left in your hair over twelve weeks because your natural hair will begin to dread around the extensions as it grows out.* If you leave them in for a longer period of time, your natural hair will break off when you have them removed.

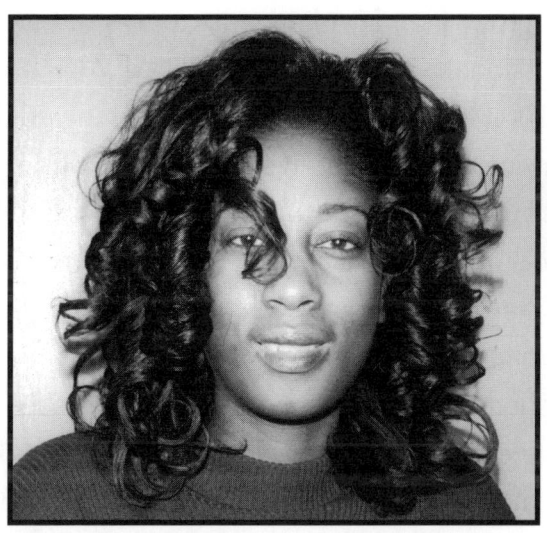

Is it her hair? You can't tell just by looking. Only her hairstylist knew for sure. Marilyn is wearing a full head of track weave, and she wears it well.

Cheryl Talley Moss

Short-Term Hair Extensions

If you do not want hair extensions to be left in your hair for a long time, you should consider having one of the short-term methods. The most popular short-term technique is called **Hair Bonding**. Tracks of hair are attached to your own hair with a hair bonding glue. This technique will only last for a few weeks because your natural scalp oil and the oily ingredients in some hair styling products will loosen the bonding glue. Hair bonding will cause hair damage if it is not professionally attached and removed. Hair bonding cost about $100.00 to $150.00 for a full head in addition to any other service you may receive. **Crochet Braids** is the hottest short-term technique out right now. The singer actress, Brandy, occasionally wears her hair extensions this way. Your natural hair is braided into vertical cornrows. Using a crochet needle, pre-braided hair extensions (usually synthetic) are attached to your cornrow braids. This service usually cost around $150.00 to $200.00. Crochet braids will last about a month. Please don't try to keep crochet braids or any other short-term hair extension method in your hair for a longer period of time because your hair will begin to look a mess. Although they can be removed at home, I recommend that a professional remove them to prevent hair breakage. Don't keep short-term hair extensions in your hair longer than recommended. Don't be cheap. If you want to keep hair extensions in your hair longer than two months, get a long-term method. It will be worth it. Think of it as an investment.

The price the hairstylist will charge for hair extensions is a good indication of the quality of the service you will receive. Top hair extension experts will include the cost of the hair into the price of the service. This is what I like to do because I don't want my clients to make the mistake of purchasing hair that is inappropriate for them. Many women purchase the wrong type of hair (human or synthetic) and the wrong color and texture that is needed for the results they are trying to achieve. If you are one of those women that like to purchase your hair for extensions, let me give you some advice: Inspect the hair carefully before you buy it. Make sure you know if the hair is human or synthetic. Human hair is more expensive than synthetic hair. You can do most of the same styles with synthetic hair as you can with human hair. It is best to use human hair for Track Weave and Hair Infusion because it will look natural longer. Synthetic hair is cheaper and is excellent for most braiding techniques. Kanekalin synthetic hair is popular because of its lightweight. If you purchase synthetic hair, be sure to get the non-flammable kind. Back in the day, synthetic hair looked like plastic; however, it is very natural looking today. If you choose to use synthetic hair for track weaving, don't leave it in longer than four weeks because it will rub against your natural hair and cause it to break off. Selecting the kind of hair you need can be very confusing. Take the hair out of the package and examine it carefully. Most beauty supply stores will not allow you to return the hair after you have purchased it. There are over a hundred different types of hair (from kinky to bone straight) to choose from. Avoid purchasing human hair that has been chemically processed (permanently waved, chemically relaxed or color treated). It will tangle easily because the hair is already damaged before you put it on your head. There are some 100% human hair types that are handpicked, strand by strand, to ensure that all of the cuticles are lying in the same direction. Note: This hair is very expensive. Your hairstylist can order it for you because it is not available in beauty supply stores. The best human hair to purchase is "French Refined." It is my favorite type of hair to work with because this type of hair is not damaged from chemical processing.

While wearing hair extensions, be sure to shampoo and condition your hair at least once a week. Don't make the mistake of neglecting your natural hair. Many women get hair extensions to give their hair a rest because it is damaged. If possible, have your hair professionally shampooed and conditioned. If you have to do it yourself, be very gentle with your hair. Don't pull on the hair extensions while your hair is wet because excessive stress on the hair will loosen them.

WIGS

Wearing a wig will allow you the opportunity to create an instant "new attitude." Wigs are simple and fun. I do not advise women to wear wigs on a regular basis unless you have a medical condition like alopecia (baldness in spots) or if your hair fell out because of chemotherapy (cancer treatment). By the way, *the major causes of hair loss for women are styling stress, genetics, and temporary situations such as illness, medication, diet, stress, pregnancy, and menopause.* Constantly wearing a wig all day long will make your hairline thinner because of the constant friction and tension to the hair in this area. Do not get into the habit of wearing a wig everyday unless you absolutely have to. Women that have healthy hair usually do not wear wigs; however, there is an exception to this rule. Sometimes celebrities or entertainers will wear wigs while they work. Excessive heat styling and studio or stage lighting can be very drying and damaging to chemically relaxed hair. One of my favorite "diva's" is Star Jones. This dynamic television personality is also an attorney, and co-host of the popular ABC morning talk show, "The View." Star often wears wigs as a fashion accessory and to protect her natural hair. And honey, she wears them well and looks absolutely gorgeous. She frequently wears her hair styled in a glamorous updo. I can see that the hair exposed around her hairline is in excellent condition, which means that her natural hair is being properly cared for. So you see, I am not totally against wearing wigs; however, I am against neglecting your natural hair while you wear them.

I personally experienced all of my hair falling out because I had chemotherapy. Being a cancer survivor has made me more sensitive to all women that must wear wigs. I open my salon early, to tend to beauty and hair care needs of clients that are bald or have thinning hair. Opening my business early allows me the opportunity to make my clients as comfortable as I can by giving them complete privacy. To have one cancer victim leave my salon with better self-esteem (while they are fighting for their life) makes getting up a little earlier well worth it.

Now, you can purchase wigs in human or synthetic hair. In the past, wearing a wig almost felt like wearing a helmet. Today wigs are constructed for comfort and are generally very light in weight. They come in a wide range of natural-looking textures and colors. Synthetic wigs are inexpensive and will keep their style for long periods of time. But remember a *cheap wig will look like a cheap wig.* Shampoo synthetic wigs in cool water with dish soap or Woolite®. Fasten the wig to a canvas wig block and set the wig as normal with rollers. Steam the wig over boiling water or a vaporizer. I recommend that you have human hair wigs professionally cleaned and styled by a licensed wig specialist or hairstylist because you can easily stretch them out of shape. If you would like to clean and style it yourself, purchase a sturdy canvas wig block, wig brush, wig comb, and glass tipped sewing pins (for setting) at your local beauty supply store. Be sure to get glass tipped sewing pins because they will not leave marks in the wig. Now you see why I recommend that you have it professionally serviced. This equipment can be extremely costly. Gently shampoo and condition your wig. Pin it to your canvas block. Roller set the wig, and allow it to dry naturally. Human hair wigs can be styled with electric rollers or curling irons. But, be sure to be very careful because if you burn the hair on the wig it cannot grow back!

Hairpieces

Attaching a wiglet or a hairpiece is also a very quick way to achieve an instant "new attitude." For a special occasion, try wearing a fall or a ponytail. For long hair that just won't quit, follow this five-step procedure:

1. Brush your hair toward the crown into a ponytail.
2. Secure your ponytail with a rubber band.
3. Wrap your ponytail into a bun to create your base, and to keep your hair in place.
4. Use bobby pins to secure your bun.
5. Now all you have to do is clip on the ponytail (or fall) and have some fun.

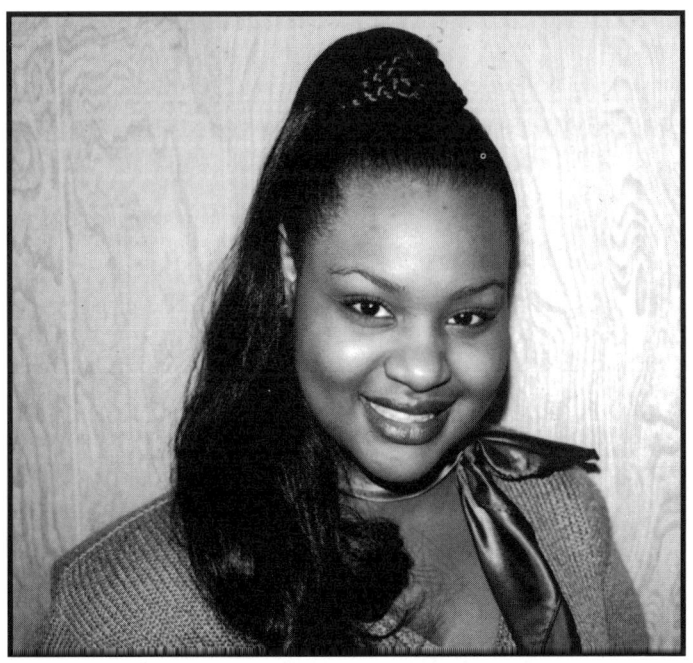

Alisa isn't afraid to wear a little "added glamour" because she knows what it takes to make a look work. So, if you like the look, go ahead and buy it, girlfriend!

It can be very easy to create various hairstyles using hairpieces. You can achieve totally different looks that can be used for daytime or evening wear.

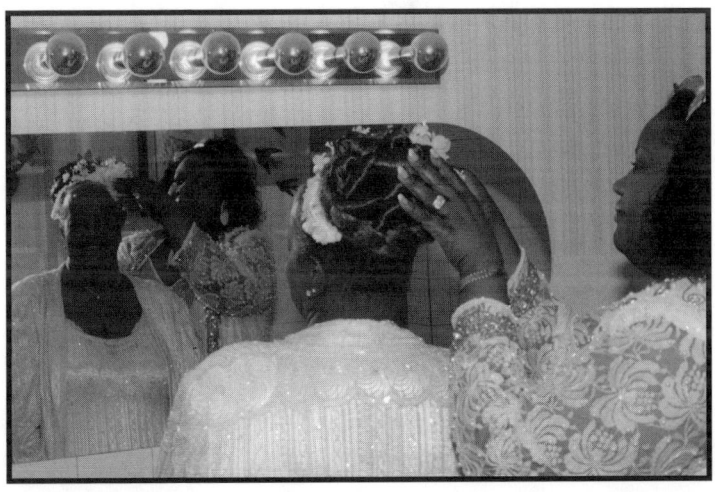

I designed this hairpiece for my mother's wedding.

Purchase your hairpiece as close to your natural hair texture as possible. Just like wigs, hairpieces come in human or synthetic hair. I prefer human hairpieces because you can change the look of the hairpiece by re-styling it. **Now sisters, please, please don't make the mistake of making a bad hair day worse by attaching a bone straight hairpiece to curly or kinky hair that is in desperate need of a retouch on the new growth of your chemically relaxed hair!**

NOTES

CHAPTER SEVEN

CHEMICAL HAIR RELAXING

Chemical hair relaxing is the process of permanently removing waves or curls from the hair. Hair relaxers are the strongest hair products on the market. **I do not recommend anyone doing his or her own chemical relaxer** treatment for this reason! Beauty industry experts say that styling versatility and convenience are the main reasons why Black women use chemical hair relaxers. **Seventy percent of all African American women wear a chemical relaxer.** More than fifty percent of all these women require a relaxer retouch every six to eight weeks. Many will attempt to do it themselves. Some women go to "kitchen-tricians" (unlicensed hairstylists that give beauty services in their home) while others have their chemical relaxer service done at a Beauty College (where cosmetology students train to become licensed) under the supervision of a licensed cosmetology instructor. But the majority of women go to a hair salon to receive the best possible service. Many women try to strip the results of the relaxer from their hair. *Chemical relaxers permanently change the inner structure of the hair.* **This process cannot be reversed.**

Now let me give you some background information on chemical hair relaxing so that you will be able to understand why **I am strongly against "kitchen cosmetology."** My mother told me that back in the 1940s there was a popular hairstyle called the "conk." This hairstyle was achieved by permanently straightening curly or wavy hair using harsh homemade concoctions of lye, potatoes, petroleum jelly, and eggs. The homemade relaxer would cause severe burns to the scalp and skin, and if it was left on the hair longer than necessary, it would dissolve the hair. My mother often reminisces about the "no pain no gain era." She can recall many stories about friends going bald or losing the majority of their hair trying to permanently straighten their hair.

In the late 1950s, before the "Afro" movement and the godfather of soul, James Brown's, popular expression, "Say it loud, I'm Black and I'm proud," hair product manufacturers started producing chemical hair relaxers. The harsh relaxers contained sodium hydroxide (lye) and required a two-step application. You had to pre-base your scalp with a light oil (that was supposed to protect your scalp) and then apply the strong relaxer to your hair. The relaxer was very thin in consistency, and it made your hair so straight that it removed the majority of its elasticity. The chemical relaxer processed very fast and left the hair in a very weak condition, which allowed it to break off easily. It also made the hair very difficult to hold any type of curls (including a roller set). Those harsh relaxers burned the scalp like hell, but Black people endured the burning process to permanently change their curly hair structure into a straight form.

Chemical relaxers improved during the 1960s; however, it was not until the 1970s that there was an innovative breakthrough. The "no-base relaxer" (that contained sodium hydroxide) was invented. Hair product manufacturers started to produce a relaxer with a creamier consistency by adding more buffers to the formula. They wanted a relaxer that would process slower and eliminate scalp burns; however, most people still received chemical burns. Throughout the years, "no base relaxers" have improved tremendously, and are considered to be the most popular type of relaxer on the market today.

Because of the explosion of the soft (jheri) curl, chemical hair relaxers were less popular in the early 1980s. Recognizing the declining use of chemical relaxers, manufacturers developed the "no-lye relaxer" to boost relaxer product sales. This type of relaxer still exists today and has gained popularity because many people are convinced that "no-lye relaxers" are better for the hair because they do not contain lye. **The simple truth is "no-lye relaxers" do contain lye.** Instead of so-called "no-lye relaxers" containing sodium hydroxide, they contain calcium hydroxide or potassium hydroxide (which are milder forms of lye). **"No-lye relaxers"** do not process the hair as fast as relaxers that contain sodium hydroxide, and they are gentler to the scalp, but they **leave the hair in a very damaged condition**. They do not flatten the cuticle enough; therefore, they leave the hair shaft wide open (without any protection) just waiting for damage to occur. After using this type of relaxer, your hair will appear to be smooth and straight; however, after about two weeks your hair will look very dull and frizzy. The hair will look under-processed and in need of another relaxer treatment. Many sisters will make the mistake of giving their hair another "no-lye relaxer" too soon trying to correct this problem, but they only end up damaging their hair even more. Manufacturers constantly come up with marketing gimmicks to trick you. They will tell you that "no-lye relaxers" are mild to the hair and will allow you to give relaxer treatments that are gentle. **Do not be fooled into thinking that relaxers that are labeled no-lye are better for your hair. I do not use or recommend anyone using them under any circumstances**.

Thank God, in the 1990s, professional sodium hydroxide relaxers are formulated to deeply condition the hair while it is being relaxed. They improve the hair's resistance to breakage because they contain conditioning agents that penetrate and remain within the hair shaft after the relaxer is rinsed out. Unlike "no-lye relaxers," **sodium hydroxide containing relaxers seal the cuticles smooth, and will give the hair an incredible sheen.**

Now let us talk about relaxer strengths because **one size does not fit all when it comes to chemical hair relaxers**. *Chemical hair relaxers come in three strengths*: *mild, regular* or *normal*, and *super* or *resistant*.

- ❖ **Mild strength** relaxers should be used on fine hair textures and permanently colored hair, and should be left on the hair for no longer than thirteen minutes.
- ❖ **Regular strength** relaxers should be used on medium hair textures, and can be left on the hair for fifteen minutes.
- ❖ **Regular strength** relaxers should also be used on coarse hair textures, and can be left on the hair for eighteen minutes.

Super strength relaxers should only be used on extremely short, resistant hair types because it is very harsh and will easily over-process the hair. Many sisters make the mistake of automatically putting a super strength relaxer on their hair if it is kinky. Kinky hair is the weakest hair type because it has the least amount of cuticles (see Chapter Two). Why would anyone put the strongest strength of relaxer on the weakest hair type? People do this because they don't know any better. I wish someone had shared this information with me when I was much younger. You see, before I attended Beauty College, I made a lot of mistakes concerning my hair. No! I need to tell it to you like it really was! I did a lot of stupid things to my hair! I guess it was my experimental stage. I have very fine, kinky hair, and I always wear some type of hair color. When I was eighteen I put a super strength relaxer on my hair. Can you guess what happened? You are absolutely right! I almost went bald from over-processing my hair. I thought you needed to put a super strength relaxer on your hair if you wanted it to be bone straight. Many women feel this way. The truth is: The straighter your hair is chemically relaxed, the weaker it will become. When you over-relax curly hair, you lose elasticity. Many women are now requesting that hairstylists don't relax their hair too straight. They want hair that has bounce and body. If you are applying a super strength relaxer to your hair please, please, please stop!!! **Only professional cosmetologists should use super strength chemical hair relaxers.**

When I owned a beauty supply store, I could hardly make a profit. I spent most of my time telling the customers about the different hair products. Because I talked too much, I blew a lot of sales. I just couldn't help myself. If a lady would come into the store to buy a relaxer kit, after our conversation, she would make an appointment to have her hair professionally done at my salon. This period in my life inspired me to write this book because it made me realize that there was a need to get the information contained in this book to the public. I eventually stopped selling beauty supplies, but it all worked out in the long run. I am sure I helped a lot of women understand why it is best to leave chemical services to professionals. If you cannot afford to go to the beauty salon often, try to have at least all of your chemical services done professionally. Ask your hairstylist to show you how to maintain your hair in between salon visits. (Be sure to read Chapter Four.)

Now let us talk about relaxer applications because there are four different types: virgin, retouch, spot, and corrective.

1. A **virgin application** is the very first relaxer treatment. The relaxer is applied to all of the hair (from the scalp area to the ends of the strand).
2. During a **retouch application** (usually every six to eight weeks,) the relaxer is applied to the new growth only.
3. When the hair is worn in an extremely short cut, approximately every three weeks, a **spot application** can be given. The relaxer is applied to the hair at the temples and the nape area.
4. When receiving a **corrective application**, the relaxer is applied where the professional cosmetologist feels it is necessary. Note: I said cosmetologist. I did not say "kitchen-trician."

Okay, I know you are wondering when I am going to tell you which relaxer brands I consider to be the best. The best relaxer systems are exclusive, professional relaxer systems that cannot be purchased "over the counter" or in beauty supply stores that are open to the general public. Professional hairstylists should use only the best hair products available. **Please do not allow any hairstylist to mix different chemical hair relaxer products together because it can cause severe hair damage.** Hairstylists are not chemists and you should not pay them for experimenting with your hair. Each product in the relaxer system is formulated for a specific purpose. For this reason manufacturers of professional relaxer product lines will not retail their products to the public and they offer training classes to *licensed cosmetologists* (usually for a fee). These classes educate the hairstylist on the importance of each product used in the system.

Any sister wearing a chemical relaxer should always take the following safety precautions. Keep in mind that I don't recommend that you give yourself a relaxer. But **if you insist on relaxing your hair, the following tips will help you.**

1. Do not apply a relaxer to your hair if your scalp is irritated or injured.
2. Wait at least forty-eight hours after your last shampoo to receive a relaxer.
3. Never brush or vigorously comb your hair before receiving a relaxer treatment.
4. Do not apply relaxer to hair that is shedding excessively or breaking off.

5. Do not apply relaxer to hair that has been treated with a soft (jheri) curl. You can go bald.
6. Do not apply a chemical relaxer to hair that has been bleached.
7. Wait at least two weeks before applying a relaxer to hair that has been permanently colored.
8. Never apply a chemical relaxer to the hair of girls under the age of nine. To do so can damage the hair severely because hair usually will not *fully* develop until little girls reach puberty.
9. Always pre-base the scalp with a light oil to prevent chemical burns (before applying the relaxer).
10. Do not apply the relaxer directly to the scalp.
11. The relaxer should be applied to the most resistant area first (which is usually the crown).
12. The relaxer should be applied to the hairline last because the hairline will process faster.
13. If the relaxer accidentally gets in the eyes, flush thoroughly with water and call a doctor.
14. Do not exceed the processing time limit.
15. When the hair is straight, rinse the hair with warm water. Never use hot water because it can cause scalp irritation, and make the hair turn back to its original curly configuration.
16. Never use neutralizing shampoo between relaxer applications. It is not suitable for weekly shampooing because it will make your hair hard and dry.

17. The most important tip I can give you concerning chemical hair relaxing is this: **For the best possible results, have your hair professionally relaxed.**

Texturizing

Texturizing is a light chemical relaxing process. It makes the cuticles smooth, while releasing a small amount of the curl in the hair. It leaves the hair in a more manageable condition. The most important concern the hairstylist has while giving this treatment is to make sure the hair is not over-relaxed to the point where the hair becomes straight. Many sisters are opting to keep their glorious curls. For this reason, texturizing is popular again. Texturized crops with a Caesar color theme in red or blonde are hot right now.

CHAPTER EIGHT

Hair Coloring

Years ago Black women that colored their hair to lighter shades than their natural hair color were labeled as "**worldly women.**" We were also called "**fast**" just because we added a little excitement to our hair color. Women of other races that changed their natural hair color to lighter shades were not labeled this way. Fortunately, times have changed. Studies show that about ninety percent of all American women wear some type of hair color and the number one reason is to cover gray.

Today hair color can be like wearing facial make up. If your skin is healthy, wearing make up can help to make you look great. The same rule applies to hair color, if you have healthy hair, coloring your tresses can make you look fabulous. **I recommend that you consult a professional hairstylist for any type of permanent hair color.** A professional hairstylist will take into consideration your hair type, texture and condition when customizing the color formula to enhance the color of your eyes, skin tone, and wardrobe. Most hair colorist are masters of illusion, and the art of color coordination. They have developed their own personal techniques to create "custom design" hair color to compliment and enhance each individual client's personality. Correcting hair coloring mistakes can be expensive, and damaging to your hair. For example, there is one hair-coloring product that should not be used on chemically relaxed hair, unless you plan to wear your hair cut very short because it can cause severe hair breakage. Now don't worry, I am going to tell you more about this product later, I keep trying to get ahead of myself. First, let us examine the different types of hair color because basically there are three types: temporary, semi-permanent, and permanent.

Temporary Hair Color

Temporary hair colors are simple rinses that **last from shampoo to shampoo.** They contain certified food colors that coat the cuticle layers of the hair. Temporary color is used on the hair the same way we use mascara on our eyelashes. The color will come off as soon as the hair comes in contact with water. Temporary hair color rinses can make your hair go darker but they cannot lighten your natural hair color. **Do not use temporary rinses to cover gray hair**; it will be a waste of time because your gray hair will still be obvious. If you perspire from your scalp, don't make the mistake of touching your hair, because temporary hair color rinses will slide right off. And don't get caught out in the rain without an umbrella wearing temporary hair color because you could soil your clothes. I personally don't use temporary hair colors because I think they are a waste of time.

SEMI-PERMANENT HAIR COLOR

Semi-permanent hair colors coat the cuticle layers and will last about four to eight weeks. They come in a beautiful array of shades that not only look great but also help to keep your hair healthy. Semi-permanent hair colors do not contain ammonia or peroxide that can damage your hair. This type of hair color will cover gray hair and will last longer when applied immediately after a chemical relaxer service because the cuticle layers lie flat and allow the color to stick better. **You cannot lighten your hair with semi-permanent hair color but you can easily go darker**. The longer the color is left on the hair, the darker the hair will become. Semi-permanent hair colors can be processed up to twenty-five minutes, but be sure to check your results after ten minutes. Since hair that has been chemically relaxed tends to be dry, using a semi-permanent hair color will help to make your hair look lustrous because the color will add a radiant shine. Semi-permanent hair color will also eliminate frizzy hair because it seals the hair cuticles.

When selecting semi-permanent hair colors, look for products that contain enriched conditioning ingredients like jojoba oil, vitamin E, and aloe vera that will actually moisturize and make the hair shine as it is being colored. Semi-permanent hair color is my favorite type of hair color to use on my Black clients. I love the way it fades naturally and allows my clients the opportunity to change their hair color frequently while leaving their hair silky, soft, shiny, strong, and healthy.

PERMANENT HAIR COLOR

Permanent hair colors are usually called tints. There are two types of tints: one-step and two-steps. Both types contain artificial color and must be combined with peroxide in order to work. They deposit color in the cortex layer of the hair and can remove natural pigment (color) at the same time. A one-step tint is applied in a single application process, while a two-step tint requires bleaching the hair first and then applying the tint. Two-step tints can be damaging to hair that has been chemically relaxed. I only recommend two-step tint applications for women that keep their hair in a "natural" style or so short that the hair that is damaged from the bleaching process will be cut off regularly. Jada Pinkett Smith occasionally wears her cropped hair this way and looks absolutely fabulous. But ladies let's not fool ourselves, everyone can't wear this bold look.

There are many different types of permanent hair coloring techniques. Highlights, streaking, chunking, and frosting are the most popular. All of these techniques involve coloring the hair in specific areas to create a special effect. Don't try any of these techniques yourself if your hair is chemically relaxed. You could cause severe damage to your hair. Kelly Shanygne Williams has admitted that she made her hair fall out because she attempted to do one of these techniques on her hair. Don't make the same mistake. Kelly was nice enough to tell the public the truth. She didn't have to. I admire her honesty, and we can all learn from her example.

The most valuable tip I can give you concerning hair color is simply this: If you want to maintain healthy (medium to long) lengths of hair, DO NOT BLEACH YOUR HAIR, if it is chemically relaxed. Bleaching chemically relaxed hair will separate the cuticle layers. Your hair will become excessively dry and frizzy, and hair in this condition will quickly begin to break off.

Be sure to leave permanent hair coloring to the professionals. Please do not allow hair color manufacturers that

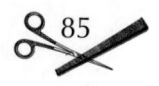

spend millions of dollars on advertising campaigns, to fool you. The Black model, with chemically relaxed, bleached blonde hair, you see on the permanent hair color box will not have healthy hair for long. Have you ever read the back of a relaxer container? If you haven't, please read one. Any relaxer container will state in bold letters: **DO NOT USE ON HAIR THAT IS BLEACHED**. As soon as the model on the hair color box gets a relaxer retouch, her hair will become over-processed and will break off. Trust me, while I was teaching Beauty School, I saw this type of hair damage all of the time. Be sure to wait at least two weeks after receiving a chemical relaxer before applying a permanent hair color.

Now let us talk about color selection. I am not going to tell you what shade of hair color you should wear because some people have the confidence and personality to pull off what other people cannot. Let me give you an example of what I mean. One of my clients (I'll call her Dana) had me to permanently color her shoulder length tresses to a medium brown shade with gold highlights. Dana is a very beautiful woman, and this shade of hair color complemented her picture perfect complexion. She loved her new hair color and was very excited about the change in her appearance when she left the salon on a Thursday night. She went to work the next day, and received many compliments on her new hair color from her co-workers; however, one person made a negative comment. Instead of letting the disapproving remarks go in one ear and out of the other, Dana came back to the salon (that same day) requesting that I change her hair color back to it's original shade. I could not talk her out of it, so I did what she wanted me to do using (non-damaging) semi-permanent hair color. The following Monday morning, Dana called the salon and left a message on the answering machine. She was in a rage because (over the weekend) the woman that made the rude comments at work had her hair colored the same shade Dana's was on Friday. Can you believe that? That was really a trip!! The moral of this story is: DON'T CHANGE YOUR HAIR COLOR TO PLEASE OTHER PEOPLE! You should please yourself. But here are some things you need to consider:

- ❖ Hair color can be bold but it should always look natural.
- ❖ As you age, avoid extremely dark hair colors like black and dark brown. Dark hair colors on mature women tend to make us look hard because every wrinkle on our face will be emphasized.
- ❖ Every age group should avoid hair color the same shade of your skin tone. The color of your face blending in with your hair color isn't flattering.
- ❖ If you select an extremely light level of hair color, be sure your complexion is clear because every pimple or scar you may have will be on display.

In the past, Black women usually would lighten their hair color in the spring, and then try a darker shade in the fall. Today Black women are coloring their hair more often, rotating bold shades with more natural ones. So, If you like the bold and trendy hair colors that are popular right now (from vibrant auburn to dazzling bronze,) I say go for it. Add just the right amount of color excitement and take your hair color to the next level, after all, it is the hottest hair accessory out.

CHAPTER NINE

How To Select A Hairstylist

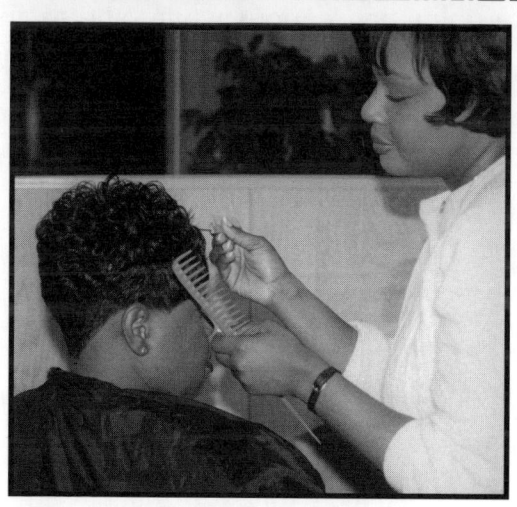

Lyndel Crosby, model. Alisa Moss, stylist.

Every good hairstylist will tell you that **word of mouth is the best form of advertisement.** Ask a sister for the name of her hairstylist if you admire her hair on a regular basis. **Do not let cheap specials lure you into a hair salon**. Salons that advertise inexpensive specials all of the time are generally cutting corners somewhere and it is usually the quality of the products they use and the quality of the service their stylists give; however, there are exceptions to this rule. Occasionally a salon will offer a special for new customers only, hoping that once the customer receives a quality service, they will return to the salon on a regular basis.

Because my hair salon is located inside of a shopping mall, women come in all of the time to check us out. You would not believe some of the weird things people do. Most women are polite and curious while others can be down right rude. If you walk into a hair salon to check it out, let me give you an example of what you should *not* do. By the way, **this is a true story**. One Friday evening around 7:30 (very close to Christmas) a lady walked into the salon and started rudely yelling at the top of her lungs. "Hey! Can any of y'all do hair good up in here?" I need to let you know that this occurred at a time when our salon was extremely busy. You see, we opened the salon at 8:30 that morning and everyone had been working non-stop. I guess one of my stylists had been rubbed the wrong way that day and decided to take matters into her own hands. She yelled back at the woman: "As you can see, everybody is extremely busy here. But to answer your question: No! All of the ladies you see in here come in every week to have their hair styled and receive bad service each time!" All of the clients and hairstylists immediately began to laugh at the lady. Needless to say, the woman left in a hurry, and you could tell that by the way she rolled her eyes that she was pissed off. Now I am not proud of this, but I have to admit to you that I joined in the laughter. I couldn't help myself! It was funny! My hairstylist's response was not professional but what can I say, except that we are all human. Later, I reprimanded her privately for making the sarcastic remarks. But I have to admit to you that I was laughing the entire time!!

When you walk into a hair salon, don't be afraid to ask questions, but try to be polite. If it is at all possible, schedule a consultation with the potential hairstylist. A consultation will allow the hairstylist the opportunity to examine your hair and to make recommendations. Be prepared to ask a lot of questions. You can learn plenty of information by asking the right things. **Some of the questions I recommend asking the hairstylist are:**

- ❖ What type of products do you use?
- ❖ What type of services do you provide?
- ❖ How much do you charge for these services?
- ❖ How far apart do you book your appointments?
- ❖ What are your working hours?
- ❖ How long have you been licensed?

Other things you should consider are:

1. The cleanliness of the salon is very important.
2. Make sure there is adequate parking.
3. Check the outside lighting (especially if you will be making evening appointments).
4. Be sure your hairstylist is neatly dressed and well groomed to make a good first impression.
5. The stylist should also have hair that is healthy and attractively styled. **If the stylist's hair is tacky looking, how in the world can he or she tell you how to care for yours?**

Tell the hairstylist the services that you are interested in receiving, and ask additional questions about those specific services. Listen carefully to the hairstylist's answers to make sure that he or she is knowledgeable on the subject matter.

How To Be A Good Client

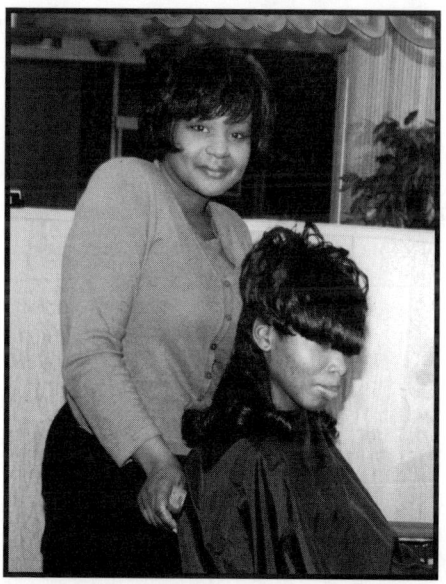

Victoria Brown, model. Alisa Moss, stylist

Now, I have told you how to select a hairstylist, let me tell you how to be a good client. Here are some of the things hairstylists love their clients to do:

❖ Always make an effort to be on time. If a client is late, it can throw the hairstylist off schedule (sometimes for the entire day).

❖ If you must cancel an appointment, call as soon as you know you are unable to keep it. This allows the hairstylist the opportunity to schedule another client in your time slot. Many stylists over-book appointments because they are afraid of clients not showing up.

❖ Be respectful of your hairstylist's recommendations.

After all, you are paying for the hairstylist's expertise. Sometimes we cannot give you what you want because it is impossible, or it may not be best for your hair.

Follow all of the rules of the hair salon. For example, if children are not allowed, don't bring them. I remember one time I had to re-schedule an appointment because my client wanted me to permanently color her hair while she held her two month old child in her arms. I would not risk the chemical dripping on her baby. If the hair color got into her child's eyes, it would have been devastating, and I would have been liable.

Last but not least, be honest with your hairstylist. If you have done things to your hair in the past, like using boxed "kitchen chemical relaxers," and drug-store permanent hair coloring, tell your hairstylist the truth. You will be surprised, the hairstylist usually can tell anyway.

CHAPTER TEN

Frequently Asked Questions & Answers

The location of my salon was very instrumental in writing this chapter of the book. I put a question box in the reception area, and over a thousand women responded. Here are the answers to your most common questions:

Q: I have a soft curl perm. Why do only a few hairstylists in my area offer this service?

A: Soft curls over-process the hair. They leave the hair in a weak, dry, and brittle condition that requires constant saturation of curl activator and moisturizer. Today, hairstylist are more professional and are into making sure that their clients hair is healthy. They are refusing to do any and every type of beauty service just to make a buck.

Q: I had a soft curl on my hair. My hair was falling out because I think it was over-processed. I had the damaged hair cut off. While I am waiting for my hair to grow out, I am wearing a wig. How should I care for my natural hair while wearing a wig?

A: Shampoo and condition your hair at least once a week. Your natural hair can be braided into small cornrows. This braiding technique will keep your wig from rising off your head. Always wear a nylon wig cap under your wig to prevent the wig from touching your skin and to keep your natural hair from slipping through your wig.

Q: My pregnant friend wants to get highlights. Could this be harmful to her unborn child?

A: This hair service is okay for the fetus according to the American College of Obstetricians and Gynecologist. If the highlights are done correctly there is no risk to the developing baby because the chemicals used to achieve the highlights are contained in the foil or paper and do not actually touch the scalp.

Q: How old should a girl be in order to receive a chemical relaxer? I put a "kiddie perm" on my five-year-old daughter's hair. Her hair is breaking off severely and she is bald around the hairline. What should I do now?

A: I know that "kiddie perms" are popular because busy parents are looking for styling convenience for their daughters. I do not recommend using them or any other type of chemical relaxer on little girls until they reach puberty (see Chapter Seven). Take your daughter immediately to a professional hairstylist for conditioning treatments. If she has bald spots, her hair is severely over-processed. Make sure that you are not contributing to the problem by putting too much tension on her weak hair. I don't recommend the use of rubber bands on little girl's hair, especially if it is chemically relaxed. It makes me upset to see a little girl with rubber bands in her hair that are so tight that there are pimples on her scalp. Try braiding your daughter's hair loosely. If the hair is braided too tight, it will cause hair loss. Be extra careful about applying too much tension on the hairline because this type of pressure will make the hair snap off quickly. Be sure to shampoo and condition your daughter's hair weekly, and wait until she is older before you let her receive another chemical relaxer.

Q: What do you consider to be the best and least expensive way to change the look of your hair?

A: A new hair cut is the most dramatic measure a woman can take to change her look, and it doesn't cost a lot.

Q: I am only twenty-four years old, and my hair is fifty percent gray. I have more gray hair than my parents. Can you tell me why?

A: Canities is the technical term for gray hair. The cause of gray hair is the loss of natural pigment in the hair. You probably have acquired canities. This condition can be premature in early adult life. The causes of acquired canities can be worry, nervous strain, anxiety, illness or heredity. If your parents didn't gray early in life, a medical condition or stress could have caused your gray hair. I recommend that you see a physician. If you are uncomfortable about having gray hair at your young age, go to a professional and have it colored.

Q: I burned my hair using a curling iron, and even after washing my hair a few times, I still smell burned hair. How can I get this terrible odor out of my hair?

A: I understand your predicament because burned human hair smells like burning chicken feathers. This awful odor will indeed stay in your hair if you do not cut the burned hair off; however, if the hair is only slightly singed you can apply an acid rinse to remove the odor. Shampoo and towel-dry your hair. Rinse the hair with tomato or lemon juice. You can also use a solution of equal parts of water and vinegar. The acid rinse usually removes the odor. If it doesn't, have the burned hair cut off. It will break off any way. Because acid rinses are drying to the hair, be sure to follow the rinse with a moisturizing conditioner.

Q: I wear extension braids. Every two months I take the braids out and have my hair chemically relaxed. Each time I remove the braids, my hair sheds a lot, and is very dry and brittle. After I remove my braids, how long should I wait before receiving another relaxer retouch?

A: You shouldn't get a chemical relaxer if you are going to wear braids on a regular basis. Your hair will braid better if it is left in its natural state. You will have some shedding when you remove the braids because **it is normal to lose up to eighty strands of hair a day**. When you take the braids out you will lose all the hair (at one time) you would normally shed daily; however, improper removal of the braids will contribute to your loss of hair. After you remove the braids (using a detangling spray and a wide tooth comb) comb the hair from the hair ends upward, instead of pulling the hair from the scalp area.

Q: I have shoulder length, thick hair, and I wear my hair thermal pressed. Over the past seven years, I switched hairstylist many times because they stopped thermal pressing hair. Why are so many hairstylists discontinuing this hair service?

A: Thermal hair pressing is a service that will temporarily straighten naturally wavy, curly, and kinky hair by using a heated straightening comb. It will not alter the inner structure of the hair, and the hair will revert to its original curly configuration in humid conditions or when the hair comes in contact with water. It is a service many hairstylists do not provide because it is very time consuming. I personally don't thermal press hair because I have seen the long-term effects. Many women that have their hair thermal pressed (especially those that have been doing it since they were children) have permanent bald spots. Because the oil (used to lubricate the hair as it is being straightened) melts and drips on the scalp causing foliculitis (burning and or infection to the hair follicles). Continuous damage to your hair follicles can cause permanent baldness. Now I'm not saying that everyone that gets their hair thermal pressed has (or will eventually get) bald spots. Queen Latifah has said that she has her hair pressed on a regular basis. Her hair looks very healthy and lustrous. I'm sure her hairstylist is taking every safety precaution to keep her scalp healthy. Most women that receive this service will get it once a month; however, I recommend that thermal pressing be done (carefully) on a weekly basis because a month is entirely too long to go without shampooing your hair.

Q: My mother's hair is falling out because of chemotherapy. Will her hair ever grow back to the way it was before the treatments?

A: I can tell you because of my personal experience with chemotherapy (and from my experience working with cancer victims) your mother's hair will grow back as her health improves. The first few inches of hair that grows back (usually) will be a little curlier and more resistant to chemical processing.

Q: Is it safe to use baby shampoo on chemically relaxed hair?

A: In order to answer your question, I must first tell you a few things about baby shampoos. They have the same pH factor (potential hydrogen) as your tears and other body fluids. This is why baby shampoos do not irritate your baby's eyes. Baby shampoos should not be used on chemically relaxed hair or any other type of chemically processed hair. It will make the hair hard because of its high pH factor of 7. You should use a moisturizing shampoo with a pH factor between 4.5 and 5.5 on all chemically treated hair. **Baby shampoo was designed to be used on what the name implies . . . BABIES.**

Q: Can you strip a chemical relaxer off of your hair?

A: Chemical relaxers cannot be stripped off of the hair. Once you receive a relaxer, there is no turning back the hands of time. Your hair structure is permanently altered. The chemical bonds inside of your hair have been permanently changed. (Read Chapter Seven.)

Q: I am a senior citizen on a fixed income, and I cannot afford to have my hair done professionally. I have a chemical relaxer on my hair but it is thinning and breaking off. Every time I give myself a relaxer, I get really bad scalp burns. What do you suggest I do?

A: Most Beauty Colleges offer a discount for senior citizens. Check out your local Beauty College. Students training to become licensed hairstylist perform the services, and the prices are guaranteed to be reasonable. Your hair is probably thinning because of your age and the fact that you are (most likely) over-processing your hair. Constantly receiving chemical burns on your scalp each time you give yourself a relaxer will also contribute to the thinning of your hair. Black women have a tendency to have keloids (scar tissue that grows over abrasions or sores). If you are burning the hair follicles (pockets of skin on the scalp that hold the hair strands) keloids can form as your scalp burns heal. If this occurs, it is a strong possibility that your hair will never grow back in that area.

Q: A few years ago I had my hair cut short. Now it seems as if my hair won't grow back. My hair grows to a certain length and stops. Can a haircut stunt my hair growth?

A: Hair growth starts from within your body. A haircut will not stunt your hair growth. You are probably caught up in the break-n-grow process (read Chapter Two).

Q: I love the way my hairstylist makes my hair look. This is my problem: Each time my hairstylist thermal curls my hair, my scalp gets burned. Should I say something to her about it?

A: Your question reminds me of an incident that occurred at a hair salon I worked in during the 1980s. This was during a time when just as many brothers would get their hair professionally blow-dried and curled as sisters. It seemed as if everywhere you turned, brothers were looking like Al Sharpton or

James Brown. Sisters, y'all remember when the brothers stayed in the mirror longer than we did. Tyrone (one of the salons clients) would get his "do" done by Pam every two weeks, and just like clockwork, each time she curled his hair, she would burn his scalp. Now, I have to give Pam credit (even though she burned her clients) she could style hair well. Tyrone's hair would always look sharp, or as the young people say today, his hair was "the bomb." I remember one Saturday in particular, Pam was burning Tyrone's scalp more than usual because each time her Marcel curling irons touched his scalp he would hiss "Ssss! Oooh! Wee!" And Pam would reply, in a sugary sweet, southern voice. "Oh, I'm sorry honey chile, it's just the hot grease." Well after burning him a few more times, Tyrone finally had *had* enough. He stood up from the styling chair, yanked his protective cape off of his neck, and started yelling at the top of his lungs. "Pam if that hot grease burns me one more time, call the damn fire department!!!" So, to answer your question: Don't continue to sit in the hairstylist chair feeling like you are waiting for the fire department to come! **By all means, say something!!!**

NOTES

Conclusion

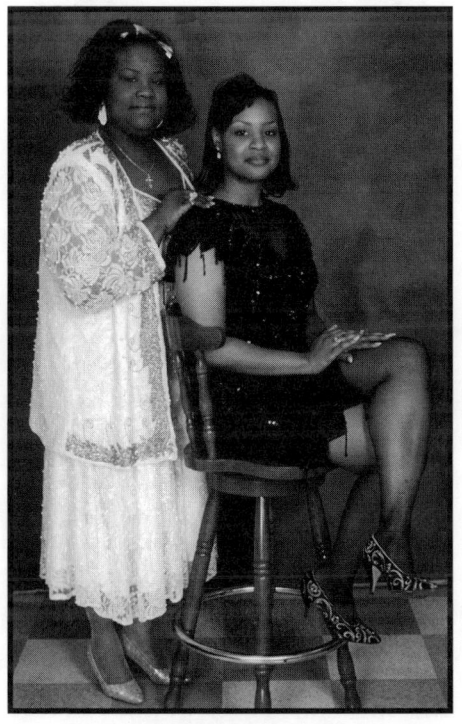

Cheryl and Alisa Moss

By the way, if you didn't guess, the hair client that was featured the most is my daughter. Alisa Latrice Moss is a business major at the University of North Texas, and is also a successful cosmetologist.

Cheryl Talley Moss

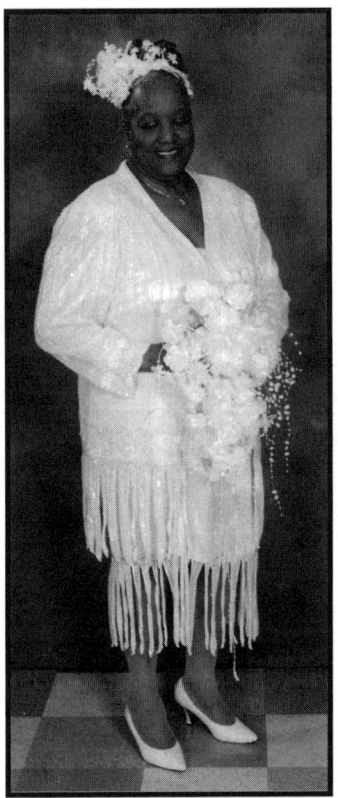

Mildred Georgia Talley

This book would not be complete without including this photo of the sweetest person I know, my mother. After being divorced for thirty-eight years, my parents remarried. But that's another book! At the time this picture was taken, Mom was almost seventy. Isn't she lovely?

We have covered a lot of hair territory, and I really hope you enjoyed the journey. But most importantly, I sincerely hope that you will begin to put some of the hair care tips into practice. Be kind to your hair and always remember that your hair is a reflection of you, and it must be nourished to remain healthy. I felt it appropriate to end this book by letting you know that I, like most hairstylists, have seen many horrible mistakes that could have been avoided. If you have made wrong hair decisions in the past, start over today and make a new beginning. Old habits are not hard to break. Honor your tresses by understanding what is best for its texture and length. Whether you prefer to have your hair chemically relaxed, or left in its natural state, whether you prefer to wear your coiffure short, medium, or long, let this book assist you in making your hair the healthiest it can possibly be. And remember everyone can have "good hair." By treasuring your crown and glory, you are sure to experience the beauty of having healthy, lustrous hair. May God bless you.

Cheryl Talley Moss

Dear Readers:

Thank you for reading this book. I would love to hear from you. If you have any questions or comments, please write me at the address below. I promise to answer any questions you may have concerning Black hair care. I look forward to hearing from you. Send a stamped, self-addressed envelope to:

Talley Publishing
c/o **Cheryl Talley Moss**
P.O. Box 870871
Mesquite, Texas 75187-0871

ORDER FORM

Please send me _____ copie(s) of

HEALTHY HAIR CARE TIPS FOR TODAY'S BLACK WOMAN

Price Per Book	$13.99
Tax Per Book	1.08
Shipping and Handling	<u>3.00</u> per book
TOTAL	$18.07 per book

Send Check or Money Order to:
Talley Publishing Company
P.O. Box 870871
Mesquite, TX 75187-0871

Name: _____

Address: _____

City: _____ State: _____ Zip: _____

Phone: (_____) _____

Please make check or money order payable to ***Talley Publishing***.
Allow 2-4 weeks for delivery.

THANK YOU!

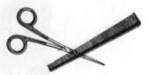

NOTES